"Dr Giroux has written an excellent book for people with Parkinson's disease, based upon her years of clinical experience, her unique insights into the patient perspective, and her extensive knowledge of integrative medicine. This book will be a 'must-read' for the many patients who are seeking a balanced, well-informed viewpoint on traditional and complementary aspects of PD care."

—*Melanie M. Brandabur, MD,*
Medical Director, Ultragenyx Pharmaceuticals

"This book is a wonderful addition to understanding the importance of integrative medicine in Parkinson disease. It lays the groundwork for a comprehensive understanding and implementation of various therapies. It is a must have for patients and practitioners."

—*Rita Gandhy MD, MPH,*
Movement Disorders Neurologist, The Parkinson's Disease Institute

"Exercise or medication alone is not enough. People with Parkinson's disease need to be empowered and educated at the stage of diagnosis with resources about what they can do to get better and stay better. *Optimal Health with Parkinson's Disease* provides a toolbox full of those resources which contain the potential to optimize brain health, symptoms, function, quality of life, and response to exercise and medication."

—*Becky Farley, PT, MS, PhD,*
Chief Executive Officer/Founder, Parkinson Wellness Recovery

Optimal Health with
Parkinson's Disease

Also by Monique L. Giroux, MD

Alter Your Course: Parkinson's—The Early Years (with Sierra M. Farris, PA-C)

DBS: A Patient Guide to Deep Brain Stimulation (with Sierra M. Farris, PA-C)

Every Victory Counts: Essential Information and Inspiration for a Lifetime of Wellness with Parkinson's Disease (with Sierra M. Farris, PA-C)

Optimal Health with Parkinson's Disease

A Guide to Integrating Lifestyle, Alternative, and Conventional Medicine

Monique L. Giroux, MD

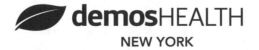

demosHEALTH

NEW YORK

Visit our website at www.demoshealth.com

ISBN: 978-1-936303-85-4
e-book ISBN: 978-1-61705-248-4

Acquisitions Editor: Julia Pastore
Compositor: Westchester Publishing Services

Medical information provided by Demos Health, in the absence of a visit with a health care professional, must be considered as an educational service only. This book is not designed to replace a physician's independent judgment about the appropriateness or risks of a procedure or therapy for a given patient. Our purpose is to provide you with information that will help you make your own health care decisions.

The information and opinions provided here are believed to be accurate and sound, based on the best judgment available to the authors, editors, and publisher, but readers who fail to consult appropriate health authorities assume the risk of injuries. The publisher is not responsible for errors or omissions. The editors and publisher welcome any reader to report to the publisher any discrepancies or inaccuracies noticed.

Library of Congress Cataloging-in-Publication Data

Giroux, Monique L., author.
  Optimal health with Parkinson's disease : a guide to integrating lifestyle, alternative, and conventional medicine / Monique L. Giroux.
      p. ; cm.
  Includes bibliographical references and index.
  ISBN 978-1-936303-85-4 (hardcopy : alk. paper) — ISBN 978-1-61705-248-4 (ebook)
  I. Title.
  [DNLM: 1. Parkinson Disease—therapy. 2. Parkinson Disease—diagnosis.
  WL 359]
  RC382
  616.8'33—dc23
                              2015030366

Special discounts on bulk quantities of Demos Health books are available to corporations, professional associations, pharmaceutical companies, health care organizations, and other qualifying groups. For details, please contact:

Special Sales Department
Demos Medical Publishing, LLC
11 West 42nd Street, 15th Floor
New York, NY 10036
Phone: 800-532-8663 or 212-683-0072
Fax: 212-941-7842
E-mail: specialsales@demosmedpub.com

Printed in the United States of America by McNaughton & Gunn.
15 16 17 18 / 5 4 3 2 1

*To my mother who shaped her own journey with chronic illness
by showing compassion and empathy for others.*

Contents

Introduction

By definition, Parkinson's disease (PD) is a movement disorder. In reality, PD is more than this label implies. Once diagnosis is made, the many non-motor symptoms become more apparent and often hold even greater significance than the movement symptoms. Motor symptoms and non-motor symptoms alike impact daily living. Coupled with this is the fact that PD is a progressive condition, which raises questions about the future.

How can I best prepare and, most importantly, what can I do to influence the future, the symptoms, of this disease?

It is so often the case that individuals living with PD, and indeed many progressive neurologic conditions, become defined by their symptoms. If symptoms are left unchecked, your life becomes the disease, with the quality of each day or moment determined by the degree or severity of these symptoms. Treatment too can focus only on symptoms, neglecting to support you as a person.

You are not your disease. But you are living with your disease. Living your best, then, means a focus that extends beyond the treatment of symptoms. It means having a broader focus that encompasses emotional adaptation, resiliency, personal healing, and prevention. You are unique not just in the symptoms you experience but also in how you approach life and live life with PD.

This book is written to help you live and thrive. It is intended to help you move beyond a reductionist and traditional approach defined by symptoms to an integrative or holistic approach. This approach respects you as a person and reinforces the concept that traditional medical therapies work best when you are empowered and supported in your quest to influence healing on an emotional, physical, and even physiologic level.

An integrative approach complements traditional medical care, which focuses on medications and surgical interventions, by introducing therapies designed to promote personal healing and well-being. In conventional or traditional medicine, these therapies or healing arts are often referred to as alternative or complementary, implying that they are somehow different in their approach or intention. These therapies are perhaps different in their focus on personal empowerment and healing, but not in their goal of better outcomes and better living.

Many physicians are leery of these approaches and sometimes for good reason. Conventional medicine and treatments are held to the principle of "evidence-based medicine." Treatments undergo aggressive testing, ideally controlling for more generalized effects such as the placebo effect. (You will learn more about this important topic as you read the chapters.) The Food and Drug Administration (FDA) regulates the use of treatments, defining the specific conditions or disease for their use and further ensuring that the benefits outweigh the risks for each therapy.

Alternative therapies are not as strictly regulated and are a multibillion dollar industry subject to strong commercial and marketing influences. Without regulation, such treatments are often promoted to treat symptoms and even cure disease without the evidence to support these claims. Anecdotal reports and personal stories touting benefit are often used to sell a product or treatment, while the results of rigorous testing and direct outcomes to support these claims are overlooked. Physicians and patients alike must navigate the truth from the hype and evaluate them with a critical eye.

This book is designed to serve as your guide, providing you with information on the role integrative medicine can play in treating PD along with a systematic approach to help ensure that your personalized care is effective and safe. With this in mind, you will first explore the philosophical underpinnings of an integrative approach, followed by the scientific evidence for its use. Well-informed, you will be better prepared to make positive lifestyle changes and critically review the many therapies available to shape your personal care.

MY PERSPECTIVE AND JOURNEY

My interest in integrative medicine began early in my career during fellowship training (specialized training in movement disorders completed after formal training obtained as a neurology resident) and is shaped daily by the stories and experiences shared by my patients during their clinic appointments. I learned from my instructors, mentors, and patients alike how stress worsens motor symptoms of tremor, dyskinesia, or freezing of gait. This observation, and indeed fact, was presented as a problem to overcome and not as an opportunity. Through the eyes of my patients I was able to shift perspective away from problems and hindrances and toward new possibilities and ideas about disease, health, and healing. The very fact that stress can worsen symptoms implies that our environment, attitudes, experiences, and emotions can and will influence PD.

Could this knowledge be used to benefit patients?

Once again the answer came from my patients. Their stories have had such a powerful influence on my own growth as a physician, and my approach to the care of people with PD, that I have included them in the hope that you too will benefit from their stories.

Although it was almost 20 years ago, I remember very clearly my first appointment with an older woman who was seeing me for the first time to discuss her treatment. She told me she had PD for 25 years, which I found remarkable and in fact did not believe since she was doing so well. We talked and I questioned her further. As her story emerged, I understood.

"What is your secret?" I asked. She responded, *"I do yoga."*

Back then, exercise was not even considered a crucial part of treatment, and I quickly understood the power of her commitment to exercise and movement. As we talked further, she revealed that yoga was of tremendous help in relieving her symptoms but was *not* her secret.

"I teach yoga to people with advanced cancer and AIDS.
This, I believe, is my secret. I benefit from the
compassion I share with others."

Of all that I have learned over the years about medications, surgery, and neurochemistry, this simple statement was, and remains, my most powerful learning experience.

Each of us has the power to heal. Our thoughts, attitudes,
and experiences play a powerful role in our personal healing.
This embrace of mind, body, spirit, and compassion is an integral
part of healing and can influence how we approach life with
disease, and perhaps the disease itself.

A few years later I was performing a consultation with an individual in advanced stages of PD. As I walked into the exam room, my first impression was of a man bent over as he sat in a wheelchair. Immediately my mind anticipated his first words, expecting to hear a long list of the difficulties he was experiencing. I had to lean in very close to hear him speak since his voice was soft and barely audible. His first words were not what I had anticipated.

"I am blessed," he said.

Again wanting to learn more, I asked him to describe why he thought this when it was obvious his symptoms and movement problems were quite significant. He looked across the room and gestured toward his family. This man was a successful businessman, CEO, and "captain of industry." Before developing PD, he spent little time with his family and poured all of his energy into his work. Parkinson's changed all that, prompting him to take inventory of his life, his priorities, and values.

"Before Parkinson's," he said, "my family would not be sitting here with me. Parkinson's has given me that—an appreciation of what is truly important to me."

He now had his family as part of his life and a new definition of what it means to be well. As a doctor, I realized from this experience that focusing on disease and symptoms alone means I will fail to see the strength that can accompany fragility, the empowerment fueled by challenge, and the compassion that can emerge in the process. From this point on my very definition of health and wellness changed.

Wellness is not the absence of disease or problems. If this were the case, wellness truly would not be obtainable. Wellness is different for each of us and includes more than just the physical symptoms we experience.

As these individuals prove, you can live well with PD. Improved well-being requires an approach broader than traditional medical treatment. Despite the importance of an integrative treatment plan, there is no clear guide to help you in this endeavor. I wrote this book to introduce you to the many therapies, lifestyle choices, and experiences that can help. Equally important is the need to present the scientific underpinnings of these therapies, along with a practical and balanced approach to help you personalize your own wellness care.

How to Personalize Your Care

This book is designed to help you expand your own personal healing and care through a coupling of traditional medicine's best offerings with complementary treatment, community therapies, and personal empowerment. It is intended to educate and raise your awareness of the many therapies and treatment strategies available to you, but is not intended to endorse or prescribe any one treatment or approach. Your personalized care is unique to you—shaped by your values, experiences, and beliefs. You will explore and perhaps challenge these ideas and values as part of your own journey in self-care. Backed by the power of this information and your own personal reflection, you will be in a better position to understand and navigate the complex world of alternative and lifestyle medicine integral to your own personal healing and work with your neurologist or health care provider to integrate these therapies into your current treatment.

This book is divided into five sections, beginning with generalized information about integrative medicine and therapies and progressing to more specific information that can be applied to your situation. You may be tempted to flip through the initial pages and focus instead on the section describing individual therapies and treatments. But remember that these treatments are merely vehicles by which true healing and well-being can occur. For this reason, information is presented first within the context of the disease and the supporting science describing how these therapies may be effective. That information is followed by a discussion of how everyday living, thoughts, and values can influence holistic care and the very outcome of these treatments. Only then are individual treatments reviewed. The book is organized as follows:

- **General Overview**

  In this section you will review basic information about PD, the philosophical underpinnings and scientific rationale as to how various therapies can be effective and integrated into your overall care, and general concepts that will help you make wise and safe decisions about the integration of traditional with non-traditional treatments.

- **General Health and Lifestyle Medicine**

  Integrative health is an active process beginning with a personal commitment to health and healing and the lifelong changes that support this commitment. This outlook is so important to health and healing that it should take precedence over any integrative therapy. With this in mind, individual therapies can then be added to support a healing lifestyle. Information on general health, especially important to people with PD, is also included since a holistic approach extends beyond the focus often given to one disease.

- **Integrative Therapies**

  In this section, you will learn about specific therapies, how they work, and the evidence for their use in PD.

- **Symptom Relief**

  Parkinson's can be associated with movement and non-movement symptoms or problems. In this section you will learn about specific ways that traditional and integrative therapies can be used in concert to treat motor and non-motor problems.

- **Personalize Your Care**

  This final section includes worksheets and tools designed to help you create a step-by-step plan for personalizing and optimizing your care.

Whether you are a true believer in alternative therapies or a skeptic, the following steps will help you expand and personalize your care to gain better health.

STEP 1: KEEP AN OPEN MIND

Begin with an open mind. An open mind means that you are not accepting of all the wonderful things that alternative therapies claim to offer or skeptical of all that traditional or conventional medicine can deliver. It means that you are open to the possibility that these treatments, when carefully chosen, can add true value to your care and how you feel.

With an open mind you will be in a position to fairly assess each therapy, beginning with an understanding of its mechanism of action, followed by the evidence that supports positive (or negative) results, and finally how the therapy fits into your own needs. Approaching each therapy in this fashion is especially helpful when conclusive evidence is not available for a specific therapy.

STEP 2: PRIORITIZE YOUR CARE

Integrative medicine opens up many opportunities for new and unique strategies designed to enhance your well-being. This can be overwhelming. Begin by prioritizing what is important to you. Focus on the symptoms or problems you wish to manage. Then review how you are currently treating these symptoms and identify any new ways or approaches you can use to manage them.

For example, first think about how each problem is impacting how you feel and your day-to-day activities. Work with your health care provider to prioritize your focus if needed. Some symptoms, such as depression, may be a priority and require a dedicated focus. Depression will affect how you feel, your motivation, and your openness to new ideas and the potential for change. Focusing on one or two problems is less overwhelming and more likely to result in successful change.

Next, think about how you will focus your treatment to combat these problems. You will learn more about specific therapies for symptoms in later sections, but remember you have a choice in how you organize your care.

- Will you rely solely on medication?
- Can you commit to lifelong results through active lifestyle changes such as exercise, diet, or stress management?
- Who will be involved in your care?
- Are your treatments balanced to include emotional, physical, and social well-being?

STEP 3: ALIGN YOUR PERSONAL LIFE PHILOSOPHY AND VALUES WITH TREATMENT

Each of us brings different experiences, cultural beliefs, personal values, and philosophical approaches that will shape health and self-care. The following questions will help you understand your own values and philosophy as related to your care choices.

- Do you believe that the lifestyle choices you make can play a role in your own health?
- Are you skeptical of non-medical therapies, relying only on prescription medications and surgery?
- Conversely, are you skeptical of prescription and surgical therapies, wishing to rely only on natural or alternative treatments even when traditional treatments are proven?
- Do you tend to seek a more active approach to your care through education and lifestyle change or a more passive approach, such as using vitamins and pills?
- Do you take vitamins, supplements, and similar pills because you believe they are the best strategy for better health?
- Are you in search of the magic pill or treatment to fix your problems?

There are no right or wrong answers. The answers are *your* answers and represent your personal care values. As you answer these questions (a survey is also included in the final section of this book, *Personalize Your Care*), think about whether there is an opportunity to expand your thoughts and ideas to include a balanced integrative approach.

STEP 4: STAY BALANCED

Balance is important to integrative medicine. By its very definition, integrative medicine balances the best of traditional medicine with the best of non-traditional therapies. Viewing these therapies as mutually beneficial is important to overall results.

Balance also refers to the activities and treatment choices you make. Is your focus on pills and supplements alone? Do you tend to focus on exercise only or do you also include healthy diet choices, stress management, and emotional health as part of your balanced care?

STEP 5: REMEMBER SAFETY

The FDA regulates prescription medications and surgical procedures to ensure that a treatment is both effective and safe. Most non-traditional therapies do not have this stringent regulatory oversight. Training, certification, and therefore quality will vary among healing specialists. In addition, the idea that natural therapies are safe is not always true. Learn how to read labels, ask critical questions about claims made, and know the certification and training associated with a therapy and/or therapist. Be sure to involve your health care provider to help you make safe choices.

STEP 6: INVOLVE YOUR HEALTH CARE TEAM

Talk to your health care provider about your interest in an integrative approach. Many physicians are skeptical of or resistant to the topic of integrative medicine. This is an obstacle but not an insurmountable one. Just as there are many ways to approach integrative care, there are many ways to talk to health care providers to gain their support and guidance. A partnership with your health care provider will help you make safe and effective choices. Tips on how to raise the topic with your health care provider are included throughout this book and in the final section, *Personalize Your Care.*

Optimal Health with
Parkinson's Disease

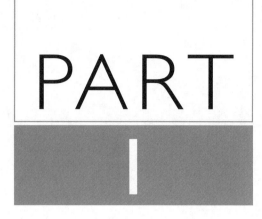

PART

I

General Overview

CHAPTER
I

Understanding Parkinson's Disease

WHAT IS PARKINSON'S DISEASE?

Parkinson's disease (PD) is a movement disorder characterized by motor symptoms of tremor, rigidity, and bradykinesia or slowness of movement. These symptoms usually begin on one side of the body and with time can spread to both sides of the body.

Motor Symptoms

The following are the primary motor symptoms associated with early PD.

Rest tremor is a rhythmic shaking noticeable in the chin or mouth, fingers, hands, arm, or leg. This tremor is present or most noticeable when the arm and leg are held in a resting or relaxed position usually while sitting, lying down, or walking. Rest tremor usually disappears or improves with activity. For instance, hand tremor is reduced with activities such as writing or eating.

Rigidity is a form of stiffness in the arms and/or legs and like tremor usually begins on one side of the body before spreading to both sides. Stiffness is noted with movement and often associated with a feeling of heaviness, tightness, or pain in the muscle. *Cogwheel rigidity* describes ratchet-like movement that can be felt when your health care provider moves your wrist, elbow, or knee during examination.

Bradykinesia is a slowness of movement that influences motor speed, initiation of movements such as first steps with walking, and motor fatigue during sequential or repetitive movements such as finger tapping.

By convention, two out of three of these symptoms must be present to diagnose PD. Tremor is the most obvious symptom often bringing patients to the doctor early in the disease, but tremor is not present in about 30% of individuals.

Postural instability describes a problem with balance experienced in more advanced disease. The problem is due to a change in the balance reflex called the *righting reflex*, which allows a rapid adjustment in posture and stance to maintain balance when the center of gravity suddenly changes, such as when stepping off a curb or stumbling over an obstacle. This reflex allows our brain to have precise control of posture and balance. When this balance reflex is diminished, unsteadiness and falls occur. These balance problems are not typical in early disease but are noted years after diagnosis.

Other motor symptoms observed as the disease progresses are as follows:

Early Stage

- Symptoms on one side of the body
- Decreased arm swing on one side when walking
- Decreased stride length or dragging the foot while walking
- Scuffing toes when walking, especially when tired
- Change in leg coordination when cycling or running
- Sense of muscle fatigue or heaviness in the arm or leg on one side of the body
- Difficulty completing repetitive movements due to muscle fatigue
- Trouble with hand coordination especially on one side, noted with bimanual tasks using both hands (such as when shampooing your hair)
- Reduced range of motion in the shoulder, shoulder pain, or frozen shoulder
- Mask-like face or a decrease in facial expression called hypomimia
- Decreased or small handwriting called micrographia

Mid-Stage

- Symptoms on both sides of the body
- Hypophonia or soft speech
- Mild swallowing problem, such as difficulty swallowing pills
- Mild flexed or bent posture and shuffling gait
- Motor fluctuations that occur when the effects of medicine start to wear off between doses
- Dyskinesia or uncontrolled involuntary movement caused by medicine

Late Stage

- Postural instability with balance problems and falls
- Freezing of gait
- Significant speech and swallowing problems
- Drooling
- Neck and trunk rigidity
- Increase in flexed posture or leaning to one side

Non-Motor Symptoms

PD is more than just a movement disorder, and indeed certain non-motor symptoms may impact quality of life more than motor symptoms. This is especially true for symptoms of depression and cognitive function. The following is a list of non-motor symptoms associated with PD. These symptoms are characterized broadly as autonomic (part of the nervous system regulating control of involuntary organ function), sensory, cognitive-behavioral, and sleep-related problems.

Autonomic Nervous System

- Constipation
- Gastric bloating and reflux
- Urinary control (frequency or urgency)
- Labile blood pressure (high and low swings)
- Orthostatic hypotension and dizziness, a drop in blood pressure when changing position from lying down to sitting or from sitting to standing
- Temperature dysregulation, such as cold hands or feet or drenching sweats

Sensory

- Pain or numbness often in arms, legs, or abdomen
- Restless legs syndrome
- Loss of smell
- Vision change, such as reduced depth perception or difficulty seeing in situations with low contrast and low lighting
- Altered taste (usually associated with loss of smell)

Cognition and Behavior

- Executive dysfunction, such as trouble with multitasking, cognitive flexibility, abstract thinking, or speed of thought
- Psychosis or, more commonly, visual hallucinations caused by medicines
- Depression

- Anxiety
- Apathy
- Daytime sleepiness
- Fatigue
- Social withdrawal
- Impulsivity problems, such as pathologic gambling or binge eating or spending, often caused by medicines
- Decreased desire to eat or increased desire for sweets

Sleep

- Restless legs syndrome
- Fragmented sleep and early awakening
- Sleep apnea
- REM (or rapid eye movement) sleep disorder (see the following list of preclinical non-motor symptoms)

Preclinical Symptoms

Certain non-motor symptoms precede diagnosis. These problems in isolation are common and not specific to PD. However, they can be the first signs of this disease, often beginning before movement problems emerge:

- Depression or anxiety, unexplained by other conditions or problems
- REM sleep disorder, defined as vivid, active, and physical dreaming, such as yelling, kicking, punching, and acting out of dreams during the REM stage of sleep
- Reduced or lost sense of smell
- Constipation

HOW DOES PD PROGRESS?

One of the most common questions I am asked is, *"How will my disease change or progress, and how quickly will it change?"* The Hoehn and Yahr rating scale identifies disease stages from mild to advanced. These stages describe motor changes that occur over time as the disease and symptoms progress.

Modified Hoehn and Yahr Rating Scale

Stage 1	Unilateral (one side of body) symptoms, minimal problems
Stage 1.5	Unilateral and axial symptoms (middle of body)
Stage 2	Bilateral (both sides of body) or axial symptoms without balance problems

Stage 2.5   Bilateral symptoms with mild postural instability (easily recovers)

Stage 3   Bilateral symptoms, mild to moderate disability with impaired postural reflexes or balance problems, but still able to walk without walker and be physically independent

Stage 4   Severely disabling symptoms, but able to walk or stand with assistance (such as use of walker)

Stage 5   Non-ambulatory, confined to wheelchair and/or bedridden

One study of 695 people showed that the average time to progress from Hoehn and Yahr stage 1 to stage 2 was 20 months; from stage 2 to 2.5 was 62 months; from stage 2.5 to 3 was 25 months; from stage 3 to 4 was 24 months; and from stage 4 to 5 was 26 months. How quickly symptoms change for you as an individual will certainly vary. Some factors such as age predict a faster decline. Depression and the presence of other medical problems are additional factors that can negatively influence physical symptoms if not the disease itself. Yet other factors under your control, such as exercise, diet, and stress management, can be associated with better health, slower change, and even symptom improvement. Your proactive approach will influence your own trajectory.

The Hoehn and Yahr scale illustrates another important point. We have clear knowledge of how symptoms can change over time. With this knowledge comes power and motivation to put a plan in place to reduce or delay anticipated problems. A focus on prevention will change the course and timeline of your disease. Speech, balance, depression, physical strength, and stamina are examples of symptoms or problems that can be targeted at any stage of the disease with the intention of improving your future.

What's more, your brain will react to these positive changes in physiologic ways that go beyond prevention. The science behind neuroprotection and neuroplasticity will be touched on in greater detail elsewhere (see Chapter 3), but the results are clear. How you live, the activities you chose, and the experiences you have will impact brain activity and how you experience PD symptoms.

WHAT CAUSES PD?

PD is associated with loss of nerve cells in a region of the brain called the basal ganglia. The basal ganglia is located deep within the brain and represents a network or interconnection of cells that work together to produce motor, emotional, and cognitive actions. The following drawing represents a vertical two-dimensional slice through the brain showing the important nuclei or group of cells that are a part of the basal ganglia. This complex network of cells is involved in the planning, initiation, learning, and execution of movement.

Nerve cells originating in the substantia nigra degenerate or die, the result of which causes symptoms of PD. These nerve cells produce an important

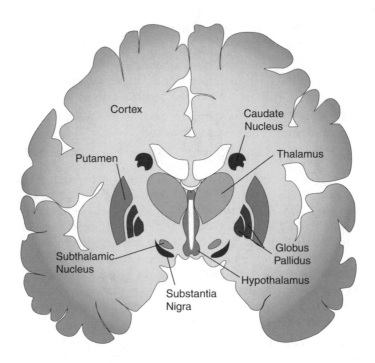

neurotransmitter called dopamine. As the nerve cells die, dopamine levels reach low levels and motor symptoms emerge.

The DaTSCAN approved for use in 2012 is a nuclear medicine brain scan that can help determine if tremor is caused by PD or other causes. This brain scan measures dopamine nerve cell levels in the basal ganglia. The following picture compares the DaTSCAN[1] image of a person without PD (left) to that seen in early-, mid-, and late-stage disease (far right). The center of each image shows the dopamine nerve cell concentration and, with PD, the asymmetry and decline that is associated with progression.

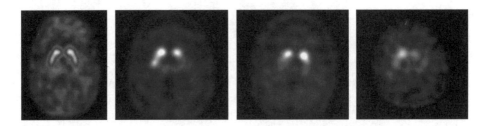

Of interest is the fact that first motor symptoms do not appear until 60% to 80% of dopamine nerve cells are lost. This fact highlights the concept of resiliency of the brain and the body's ability to compensate for and limit symptoms even

---

[1] Image courtesy of GE Healthcare.

when change with disease is significant. This ability to modify symptoms in the face of disease is an important tenet of integrative medicine. In other words, are there activities or treatments that can reduce or enhance resiliency and therefore exacerbate or improve symptoms for a person? Although science has not yet provided definitive answers to this question, epidemiology (the study of large populations to define patterns, risks, or factors associated with disease) provides clues to suggest this is indeed the case.

Epidemiologic studies offer significant clues about factors associated with an increased risk of PD and therefore possible causes and/or avenues of therapy. Some of the strongest evidence to date suggests that exposure to known environmental toxins such as pesticides and industrial solvents, such as those used in industrial agriculture and the dry-cleaning industry, are associated with an increased risk of PD. Conversely, lifestyle factors such as a prudent diet (a diet high in fruit, vegetable, and fish intake) and exercise can reduce the risk of developing PD.

Once risk factors are identified, the next step is to gain a better understanding of how these factors affect brain chemistry, physiology, and disease. Neuropathological studies bring into question the original teaching that PD is caused solely by dopamine nerve cell loss in the basal ganglia. Although this is true, it does not tell the whole story. The Lewy body is the pathological feature defining PD at the cellular level. The Lewy body is an abnormal protein deposit found in nerve cells of people with PD. Pathological studies analyzing Lewy body deposition at autopsy show the first signs of nerve damage and Lewy body deposits in the olfactory bulb (nerve cells in the nose) and the nerves along the gastrointestinal tract. These changes are noted long before the first signs of cell damage and loss are measured in the brain and may, in part, explain the presence of the many associated non-motor symptoms. But these findings also suggest a more interesting phenomenon—the first signs of PD are located in areas of the body and nervous system directly exposed to the environment. Although only speculation, could it be possible that specific environmental exposures trigger a chain of chemical reactions in nerve cells in people who are at risk for PD?

Indeed, if toxins and other environmental exposures increase risk of disease, can their exposure or effects be minimized to prevent or treat disease? This is a guiding principle of integrative medicine. The following examples illustrate how this can occur.

Oxidative Stress. Certain pesticides are linked to dopamine nerve cell damage similar to that seen in the substantia nigra in PD. Toxicity occurs through oxidative stress, a process discussed in greater detail in Chapter 3. An integrative medicine approach tackles this problem in these ways:

- The first is to limit exposure to pesticides by choosing pesticide-free produce or organic foods, if possible, and by encouraging gardeners to limit chemicals in their own gardens and/or household.

- The second is through a diet high in antioxidants, to combat overactive free radicals and the unchecked oxidative stress lethal to nerve and other cells.

- Third, prescription medicines and supplements are studied using laboratory and animal models of PD to look for a treatment that blocks the chemical and cellular damage caused by these toxins.

- Finally, integrative medicine does not differentiate among lifestyle, complementary, and traditional medical therapies but promotes the idea that these therapies and changes can work together synergistically. Diet, environmental exposures, and pills could be used together to prevent exposure, block oxidative stress, and prevent or limit disease.

Inflammation. Studies suggest that inflammation plays a role in propagating neurologic changes associated with PD. Interestingly, the use of non-steroidal anti-inflammatory drugs (NSAIDs) such as the common medicines ibuprofen and naproxen used to treat pain, are associated with a lower risk of PD and even other neurodegenerative diseases such as Alzheimer's disease. Yet taking anti-inflammatories when they are not needed carries significant risk, including bleeding and kidney and heart disease. Integrative medicine offers a safe and healthier approach

- Reduce inflammation through a change in diet by limiting foods high in glycemic load and inflammatory fats (see Chapter 5).

- Consider the use of anti-inflammatory supplements (see Chapter 6).

- Explore other therapies that might reduce the body's inflammatory response, such as mind-body therapies.

- Adopt the premise that some of these therapies will not have the full body of support to prove they work to reduce brain inflammation. Until this information is available, a risk/benefit analysis can be applied to the use of these therapies. For instance, theoretical evidence suggests that mind-body therapies may reduce inflammation through their impact on immune health and production of inflammatory chemicals. But evidence to date fails to support a direct link between specific mind-body therapies and brain inflammation. However, risk is low and the potential generalized benefit is high, including mood, stress, sleep, heart, and pain benefits.

Nature vs. Nurture

Since conclusions based on epidemiologic and environmental studies are drawn from observations of very large groups of people or geographic regions and statistical analysis of probability, it is often difficult to apply this information to you as a single individual. This is especially true since multiple factors in combination with genetics appear to work together to cause PD. This is called the *multiple hit hypothesis* because factors taken individually do not necessarily cause disease, but together their contribution to disease is greatest. For instance, toxic effects of pesticides are stronger in individuals found to have certain genetic abnormalities.

In the majority of cases, genetic abnormalities do not actually cause PD but instead increase susceptibility or the risk of developing the disease. Both nature and nurture, then, come together as a combination of genetics and environment combine to increase a person's risk.

Familial or genetic PD (when a parent, sibling, or child also has the disease) accounts for only 10% to 15% of cases. Not all associated genes have been discovered, but familial cases to date are most commonly associated with these genetic mutations: LRRK2, PARK2, PARK7, PINK1, or SNCA. Most cases, however, are sporadic, likely resulting from a complex interaction between environment and genetics not yet identified.

Research suggests that genetics is more likely to play a role in people with symptom onset prior to age 40. A recent study found that 16% of people diagnosed before age 40 have abnormal genes with the most common being Parkin, LRRK2, and glucocerebrosidase. Having one family member with PD also increases risk. For example, the cumulative lifetime risk of developing PD for a first-degree family member (parent, sibling, or child) in the United States is between 3% and 7%. This is compared to a lifetime risk of developing PD of 1% to 2% in the general population.

The fact that genetics does not tell the whole story is important to integrative medicine and to you. Simply knowing that there are environmental and lifestyle factors that influence risk of disease means that there are specific changes you can make to influence this risk, even if you have the genetic abnormality.

References
Parkinson's Overview

Braak, H. 2003. "Staging of brain pathology related to sporadic Parkinson's disease." *Neurobiology of Aging* 24: 197–211.

Elbaz, A., et al. 2002. "Risk tables for parkinsonism and Parkinson's disease." *Journal of Clinical Epidemiology* 55: 25–31.

Hoehn, M., and M. D. Yahr. 1967. "Parkinsonism: Onset, progression, and mortality." *Neurology* 14: 427.

Jankovic, J. 2008. "Parkinson's disease: Clinical features and diagnosis." *Journal Neurology, Neurosurgery, and Psychiatry* 79: 368–76.

Seifert, K., and J. Wiener. 2013. "The impact of DaTSCAN on the diagnosis and management of movement disorders: A retrospective study." *American Journal of Neurodegenerative Disease* 2: 29–34.

Shulman, L., et al. 2001. "Comorbidity of the non-motor symptoms of Parkinson's disease." *Movement Disorders* 16: 507–10.

Weintraub, D., et al. 2004. "Effect of psychiatric and other non-motor symptoms on disability in Parkinson's disease." *Journal of the American Geriatrics Society* 52: 784–88.

Wu, Y., et al. 2011. "Preclinical biomarkers of Parkinson's." *JAMA Neurology* 68: 22–30.

Zhao, Y., et al. 2010. "Progression of Parkinson's disease as evaluated by Hoehn and Yahr stage transition times." *Movement Disorders* 25: 710–16.

Nature vs. Nurture

Goldman, S. M. 2014. "Environmental toxins and Parkinson's disease." *Annual Review of Pharmacology* 54: 141–64.

Kann, M., et al. 2002. "Role of parkin mutations in 111 community-based patients with early-onset parkinsonism." *Annals Neurology* 51: 621–25.

McInerney-Leo, A., et al. 2005. "Genetic testing in Parkinson's disease." *Movement Disorders* 20: 1–10.

Piccini, P., et al. 1999. "The role of inheritance in sporadic Parkinson's disease: Evidence from a longitudinal study of dopaminergic function in twins." *Annals of Neurology* 45: 577–82.

Warner, T., and A. Schapira. 2003. "Genetic and environmental factors in the cause of Parkinson's." *Annals of Neurology* 63: 818–26.

CHAPTER

2

Treating Parkinson's Disease

MEDICAL THERAPIES

To date, most medicines used to treat Parkinson's disease (PD) motor symptoms influence dopamine levels and availability at nerve synapses. The illustration on the next page shows how dopaminergic medicines can work together to increase or enhance declining dopamine levels in the brain.

Let's review the most commonly used medicines and their effect on the body.

- *Levodopa.* This medicine enters dopamine nerve cells and is chemically transformed to dopamine. One of the oldest medicines used for PD, levodopa is still one of the most effective. Essentially, levodopa will restore inadequate levels of brain dopamine, improving movement symptoms. Levodopa is combined with carbidopa (the combination is called carbidopa/levodopa or goes by the trade names Sinemet, Parcopa, and Rytary). Carbidopa prevents levodopa conversion to dopamine outside the brain, both reducing nausea as a side effect and allowing more levodopa to enter the brain where it is needed.

- *Dopamine Agonists.* This group of medicines is chemically similar to dopamine, interacting not at the dopamine nerve cell but at the adjacent nerve cell, essentially activating this cell via chemical receptors. Examples

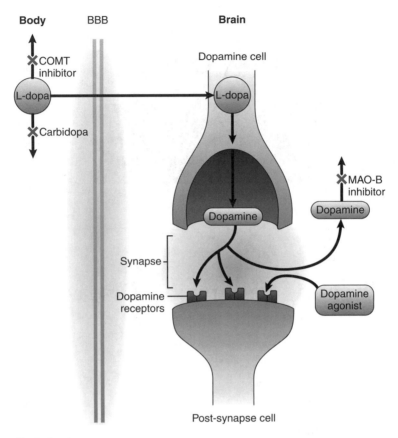

Body   BBB   **Brain**

COMT
inhibitor

Dopamine cell

L-dopa   L-dopa

Carbidopa

MAO-B
inhibitor

Dopamine

Dopamine

Synapse

Dopamine
receptors

Dopamine
agonist

Post-synapse cell

Brain Anatomy
BBB – Blood-brain barrier. Protective covering that surrounds the brain. Drugs must
     cross the BBB to enter the brain.
Synapse – Space between two nerve cells.
Dopamine receptor – Protein on nerve cell. Where drug attaches to receptor.

Drugs
L-dopa (levodopa) – Converted to dopamine in a nerve cell.
Carbidopa – Blocks L-dopa breakdown in the bloodstream.
COMT inhibitor – Blocks L-dopa breakdown in the bloodstream.
MAO-B inhibitor – Blocks dopamine breakdown in the brain.
Dopamine agonist – React directly to activate dopamine receptor.

of dopamine agonists used in the United States are ropinirole (Requip),
pramipexole (Mirapex), and rotigotine patch (Neupro). Apomorphine
(Apokyn) is a unique dopamine agonist that is injected under the skin.
This medicine is quickly effective and is used as a rescue treatment, bridging the gap between standard medication dosages when wearing off and
when end-of-dose reemergence of symptoms is a problem.

- *MAO-B Inhibitors.* Monoamine oxidase type B (MAO-B) inhibitors block
  dopamine metabolism, essentially slowing the breakdown of dopamine in

the brain and further enhancing dopamine effectiveness by elongating the time dopamine is available and active in the synapse. Examples of MAO-B inhibitors include selegiline (Eldepryl, Zelapar) and rasagiline (Azilect).

- *Catechol-o-methyl-transferase (COMT) Inhibitors.* COMT inhibitors also block the metabolism or breakdown of dopamine both in the bloodstream (entacapone, Comtan, Stalevo) and in the brain (tolcapone, Tasmar). These medicines are used with levodopa to treat the wearing-off effect at the end of dose and are therefore used in mid-stage and advanced stage disease when this problem emerges.

- *Amantadine.* Amantadine is unique in its chemical effect as this medicine is believed to enhance the release of dopamine at the synapse and block the effects of the neurotransmitters acetylcholine and glutamate. These additional properties are most likely responsible for the anti-tremor and anti-dyskinesia properties attributed to this medicine.

Medicine Pros and Cons

The decisions to start medication and which medication to use are individualized ones based on symptom severity, side effect risks, activity or occupational needs, a person's philosophical views on medication, and cost. If you are reading this book, you are interested in an integrative approach, pairing medicine with the best lifestyle and wellness therapies to achieve the best benefits. An integrative approach does and should include traditional medicines when appropriate. Medication, when used wisely, remains the most effective treatment. Only using natural therapies, without medication, may even prove harmful for the following reasons:

- Untreated motor symptoms limit activities such as exercise that are important to future health.
- Untreated symptoms cause other problems such as pain, depression, or falls.
- Untreated symptoms set up abnormal patterns of movement and habits that are hard to reverse.
- The positive benefits of natural therapies alone may not be as great. For example, the quality of movement during exercise is an important factor that influences positive brain change. Exercising more but with poorer performance may not have the same benefits.

Side Effects. All dopaminergic medicines share similar side effects:

- Nausea and vomiting
- Heartburn
- Confusion (more common with agonists and amantadine)
- Hallucinations (more frequent with agonists and amantadine)
- Sedation, daytime sleepiness, sudden sleep attacks (may be more common with agonists)

- Impulsive or compulsive behaviors such as excessive gambling, overeating, and hypersexuality problems (may be more common with agonists)
- Leg swelling (especially amantadine and agonists)
- Light-headedness or dizziness (more common with agonists and amantadine)
- Insomnia (more common with selegiline)
- Constipation, memory loss, blurry vision, dry eyes, dry mouth, and bladder retention (amantadine)
- Diarrhea (entacapone, Comtan, Stalevo tolcapone, Tasmar)

Some of these side effects are also symptoms of the disease, further complicating therapy. Integrative therapies can be very effective in mitigating some of these symptoms and side effects. Part IV is dedicated to these symptoms or side effects and potential integrative therapies.

SURGICAL THERAPIES

Deep Brain Stimulation

Deep brain stimulation (DBS) is a surgical treatment in mid-stage disease recommended to treat motor fluctuations such as medicine wearing off and dyskinesia or medicine-induced uncontrollable movement. DBS is sometimes performed in an earlier disease stage when tremor and dystonia are problems and refractory to medical therapy.

The surgical procedure involves implanting tiny wire(s) into regions of the brain that are part of the basal ganglia circuit that both controls motor function and is impacted in PD. These wires have four small electrodes that deliver customized continuous electrical impulses to specific brain sites. The following figure shows

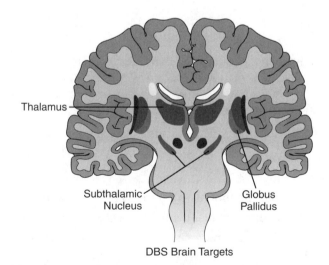

DBS Brain Targets

the three common targets for DBS electrical stimulation: the subthalamic nucleus, the globus pallidus, and the thalamus. Selection of the best target is a complex decision based on an individual's unique symptoms, medications, and surgical goals.

You will remember that in a specific region of the basal ganglia, dopamine nerve cells degenerate or die. Resultant changes in the electrical firing of neurons located in this complex circuit of nerve cells are associated with PD motor symptoms. Stimulation of these areas helps to normalize these abnormal patterns of nerve activity.

A neurostimulator (also called battery or generator) is usually implanted under the collarbone and is connected to the brain electrode wires to provide the power to send the impulses along the wire. The electrical impulses can be programmed at an outpatient appointment in the clinic through a telemetry device placed over the skin.

Although DBS is the most invasive therapy for PD, it is also the treatment most closely aligned with an integrative and patient-centered approach. This is because DBS is most effective when performed as a team approach, combining the expertise not only of neurologists and neurosurgeons but also neuropsychologists specialized in the assessment of cognitive and emotional symptoms, as well as DBS programmers and rehabilitation specialists such as physical therapists who will be treating you after surgery. The patient and family are also an important part of this team to best ensure that patient wishes and expectations are met with surgery. Hence a team approach capitalizing on the unique perspective and expertise of individual specialists and the patient is critical to outcomes.

A review of real patient discussions (obtained from patient care appointments) about DBS as a treatment option brings to light the role of patient values and biases in care that impact treatment decisions. I am in a unique position as a neurologist specializing in movement disorders and integrative medicine to observe the following phenomenon. Some patients are highly interested in natural therapies at the exclusion of pharmaceutical medicines. Yet some of these individuals seek DBS therapy earlier to avoid traditional medical therapy, believing that surgery is better (less toxic with a higher cure rate) than medication. Early DBS surgery carries additional and more serious risk, and its outcomes are much more variable and based on many more factors. In addition, DBS only matches the effect of medicines when motor fluctuations are not an issue (tremor is a noted exception) and therefore it does not bring added benefit over medicine when performed early. In this situation the risk/benefit ratio for DBS vs. medicine does not support DBS, yet DBS is still deemed more acceptable to some individuals. This situation reinforces the importance of reviewing how your fears, values, and perceptions influence your treatment choices, outcomes, and risks.

As noted, the role of the patient in the DBS process is very important before surgery but is equally important after surgery. DBS therapy significantly improves duration of medicine effect and reduces symptoms such as tremor and dyskinesia. For some, DBS can "set the clock back," reversing symptoms to the level experienced years earlier. Yet some symptoms such as speech, mood, and cognition do not improve with DBS and will increase as the disease progresses. Integrative therapy and its philosophical approach to care is especially important after DBS therapy:

- After therapy, you are feeling better, the medicine effect is lasting longer, and medicine and associated side effects may be reduced. Hopefully your motivation to enhance your care and ability to actively participate in activities such as exercise also increase.

- DBS allows you to take advantage of the fact that you are feeling better and channel this well-being into a preventive lifestyle program to reduce the onset or impact of certain symptoms, such as imbalance, which are less responsive to DBS therapy.

- DBS may in some ways simplify care by simplifying medicine dosing, but it should not be seen as a panacea designed to fix all problems going forth. DBS will not treat all symptoms, and early dramatic results do not protect against symptom decline due to disease progression and non-motor symptoms.

- Depression, even suicide, can increase after DBS even when motor symptoms are improved. Mood and well-being, then, are defined by more than physical symptoms, and treatment needs to be tailored to these potential problems.

INTERVIEW WITH THE EXPERT: DBS

A DBS EXPERT FINDS NEW HOPE AND NEW OPPORTUNITY AFTER DBS

Why is an integrative medicine approach important to people with DBS?

DBS is a surgical treatment for PD when medications or other therapies cannot maintain control of symptoms or when medication side effects become disabling or intolerable. DBS is a surgical treatment that involves implanting electrodes into specific regions deep in the brain. The electrodes supply constant high-frequency stimulation over the patient's lifetime and continues to work as long as the stimulation is adequately managed. A major benefit of DBS is the opportunity to reduce medications and related side effects. Less medication is needed

(continued)

INTERVIEW WITH THE EXPERT (*continued*)

since stimulation improves many movement and muscle symptoms.
However, the day of implantation is just the beginning.

Are there symptoms less responsive to DBS that cannot be treated with this approach?

PD symptoms cause frustration and can interfere with the simplest
activities that bring the most satisfaction in life. PD symptoms can
influence every moment, sparing little energy for activities that improve
and maintain health and happiness. For instance, tremor can change
what you eat and disrupt rest or sleep. Dystonia, or feeling "off," can
limit physical activity. Dyskinesia can wear down joint surfaces leading
to pain and decreased activity. Stimulation works well to control
stiffness, tremor, slowness, and muscle cramps and reduce dyskinesia.
However, not all PD symptoms improve with stimulation. Symptoms
that do not respond well, if at all, to stimulation include speech, mood,
cognition, bowel, and balance problems. Stimulation also does not
offer direct benefit in nutrition or fitness.

We know the immediate reaction to stimulation improves tremor,
muscle stiffness, and slowness, but we know little of the long-term
impact on disease progression when an integrative lifestyle is embraced.
Research shows us that walking, balance, and cognition typically
continue to progress despite stimulation. Yet research also shows us
that moderate targeted physical activity, stress reduction, brain nutrition, and social activity can influence mobility and cognition.

Patients who choose DBS are given hope for a new chapter in their
lives. My patients typically say DBS rolls the clock back 10 years. Individuals can prioritize daily activities to take back control of their lives. Fewer
symptoms mean more opportunity. DBS improves not only movement
and motor symptoms, but can sometimes improve fatigue, sedation,
mood, sleep, and concentration. By controlling movement symptoms and
improving sleep quality, an individual may be able to regain or maintain
the active and social lifestyle that was difficult to do before surgery.

Are there examples from your practice that exemplify this approach?

My most memorable patient that elected to have DBS was a man
in his forties. A stay-at-home dad, he was charged with getting his

(continued)

INTERVIEW WITH THE EXPERT (continued)

daughter to school and managing the household. He described his morning:

> *I wake early to crawl to the bathroom and take my pills. It takes me an hour and a half to get moving. I know I only have one hour left to take my daughter to school before the symptoms start coming back and I can't walk. My body starts to rock-and-roll as the medication kicks in. I want DBS so I can have a little more time to take my daughter for ice cream after school instead of getting home just in time to start crawling on the floor, waiting for the medication to start working again.*

This story ends well. After DBS my patient was given double the amount of time to accomplish his daily activities that now included time for exercise, healthy cooking, and hobbies, and his downtime was never as severe as before DBS.

Although a powerful therapy, DBS works best if partnered with an integrative medicine and lifestyle approach. To make the most of the new beginning after DBS, individuals can refocus their energy on a complete lifestyle makeover that includes the mind, body, and spirit for the best possible life.

Sierra Farris, PA-C, MPAS, MA, CES
DBS Program Director, Movement & Neuroperformance
Center of Colorado

Sierra is a physician assistant and expert and national educator on DBS therapies. She is also a Clinical Exercise Specialist with certification through the American College of Sports Medicine.

THE ROLE OF INTEGRATIVE MEDICINE AND DIFFERENT MODELS OF CARE

Reduction of motor problems, non-motor symptoms, and disease progression are primary goals of treatment. Medical therapies have side effects, and some side effects are similar to PD symptoms. This can sometimes limit medical therapy, requiring other means of control. In addition, concerns associated with living with a progressive condition that effects performance of daily activities can add stress and emotional distress to patients and families. The emotional, cognitive, physical, and personal impact of this disease, coupled with the many disease-influencing lifestyle and environmental factors now identified to impact risk, highlight the importance of an integrative and holistic approach. Medication, surgery, lifestyle, environment, personal and emotional healing become mutually important treatments working together to improve outcomes.

Medical care is evolving with a growing trend toward patient-centered and personalized care that reflects the true needs of the individual. With this evolution comes a parallel change in both society's and health care's acceptance of non-traditional therapies—and the very definition of medical care itself. Before we go any further, it's important for you to understand a few basic definitions of health care models and care philosophies, after which you'll get a more in-depth review of the Integrative Care Model. This information will help you navigate the complex and ever-changing health care system in the United States.

Traditional "Western" Medicine

Traditional or Western medicine is defined as a system of care to treat symptoms and disease using drugs, radiation, or surgery validated through scientific investigation. The Food and Drug Administration (FDA) and medical societies use evidence-based medicine to evaluate the appropriateness and safety of treatments for symptoms and disease, thus overseeing and ensuring the safe and appropriate use of medication, biological products, and medical devices. Evidence-based medicine supports the use of sound scientific evidence obtained through use of vigorous study methods, coupled with clinical experience and patient values to guide treatment decisions. In practical terms, evidence-based medicine does not overrely on individual case studies or stories of treatment benefits, as these can be influenced by factors unrelated to the treatment, such as marketing forces, personal expectations, and biases of clinician and patient. Evidence-based medicine places emphasis on the strongest data and results obtained through research methods that link treatment effects directly to the therapy itself. Examples of research methods that meet this criterion are the randomized controlled trial design and meta-analysis of multiple studies using stringent methods to investigate an overarching effect. Randomized controlled clinical trials control for the placebo effect, which is an important factor influencing treatment outcomes.

Critics of traditional medicine claim that evidence-based medicine is "cookbook medicine," does not take into consideration the individual needs of the patient, and focuses on disease not prevention. This is not the case as traditional medicine continues to evolve with a focus on best outcomes and safe practice. Dr. David Sackett, a known leader in evidence-based medicine, stated over 20 years ago in an article for the *British Medical Journal* that "the practice of evidence-based medicine means the practice of integrating clinical expertise with the best available external clinical evidence from systematic research."

Despite criticism of traditional medicine's shortcomings, this definition encompasses the goals and intentions of integrative medicine. The difference is perhaps integrative medicine's overarching focus on the treatment of the whole person, including disease and wellness, rather than treatment that is restricted to symptoms or disease.

Complementary and Alternative Medicine

These practices embrace healing therapies not necessarily used in conventional medicine yet supported by historical observations and cultural traditions rather than scientific measures. The National Center for Complementary and Integrative Health (NCCIH) defines this branch of medicine "to mean the array of health care approaches with a history of use or origins outside of mainstream medicine." According to the NCCIH, "complementary generally refers to using a non-mainstream approach together with conventional medicine. Alternative refers to using a non-mainstream approach in place of conventional medicine."

The NCCIH has proposed a classification of complementary and alternative therapies (CAM), a modification of which is used in this book.

- *Lifestyle Medicine.* This term encompasses the personal habits and lifestyle choices that impact health, such as sleep, alcohol and tobacco use, nutrition, exercise, and stress management.
- *Biological Therapies.* These therapies include plant-derived chemicals and products, vitamins, and nutritional supplements.
- *Body Therapies.* These therapies focus on body alignment, musculoskeletal health, physical sensations, and body movement.
- *Mind-Body Medicine.* These therapies focus on the interaction between mind, body, social, mental, and spiritual factors that promote health, heal, and enhance therapeutic outcomes.
- *Energy Medicine.* Energy medicine works with the premise that energy of many forms exists in and outside the body. When this energy is in balance, it can be used to heal; when out of balance it can cause disease.
- *Whole Medicine Systems.* These beliefs are often centuries old and based on the premise that the body is a complex interdependent system. The health of a single organ (i.e., the brain) requires that the body (at the cellular, chemical, or energy level) and organ systems function best when in harmony with our emotions, mind, spirit, community, and environment.

Patient-Centered Care

Patient-centered care is the cornerstone of modern-day chronic care management and introduces a philosophy of care that incorporates the patient experience into the treatment and planning process. This model of care is now embraced by mainstream medicine, leading to significant changes in how care is delivered (Institute for Healthcare Improvement, www.ihi.org). Patient-centered care was designated and endorsed by the Institute of Medicine in 2001 as a model of care to empower patients; improve quality of life, treatment outcomes, patient satisfaction, and efficiency; and lead to more effective medical team performance and care delivery. Patient-centered care is a system of treatment designed around the needs of the person or patient. Person-centered care is more than just offering convenient treatment; it is a philosophy of care that puts you, the patient, *front and center.*

So what exactly is patient-centered care? How is it really different from other forms of care and why is this model important to integrative medicine?

Patient-centered care involves individuals and their families in all aspects of care and care decisions. In this type of care you are the captain of your medical team. Patient-centered care is based on certain philosophical principles: Care should be individualized, actively include the patient in treatment decisions, and respect the values and relationships important to the patient when making these decisions.

Individualized Care. Each person is different, having a unique set of strengths, goals, dreams, and approaches to problems and preferences. Ideally, your treatment should include these personalized values and align with them when possible.

Participatory Care. As an active medical team member, you as the patient have the right to be involved in health care decision making and treatment. You are part of the decision to begin a treatment and ideally should understand what it can and cannot accomplish. You can help decide if a treatment is important or the *best fit* for you. As a patient of mine once said,

"I feel best when I am part of the solution!"

You are part of the solution through your participation in medical and surgical decisions and your involvement in self-care, lifestyle, and personal change that is designed to enhance your health and well-being.

Personal Value. Your cultural upbringing about your health plays a significant role in your treatment. Many people with PD carry the firm (and accurate!) belief that they do indeed have the power to heal and influence the course of their disease with a focus on different healing-based creative arts and spiritual and nature-based therapies.

Relationships. We do not live alone. Relationships are an important part of life. Relationships can be the connection to family or friends. For some, these relationships may differ and may include connections to animals, pets, one's home, community, religion, or spiritual self. Optimal care will respect and possibly include these people and/or relationships in treatment decisions.

Patient-centered care works. Many PD studies evaluating factors contributing to quality of life find that symptoms such as depression, cognitive decline, and falls negatively impact quality of life. Some of these symptoms are difficult to treat and simply suggest quality of life is tied to disease progression. Yet improved quality of life in PD is also tied to the person's sense of control and hope, as well as the quality of the clinician therapeutic relationship. This finding is very important since the quality of health care delivery and the effects of a positive therapeutic relationship can be promoted and effective throughout all stages of disease.

Integrative Medicine

Integrative medicine combines conventional medicine with therapies designed to address the whole person, promote healing, and encourage a wellness approach to preventive care and illness. This is patient-centered to the highest level and holistically designed to respect the patient's own care values, culturally based healing systems or beliefs, and use of less traditional yet validated alternative therapies. Through integration, these therapies can promote and enhance the healing effect of traditional medicine.

INTEGRATIVE THERAPIES

The use of CAM is common and of particular interest to people living with chronic or disabling conditions. Up to twothirds of the population will seek alternative medical treatments, making this one of the fastest-growing areas of medicine.

True measures of CAM use are difficult to obtain and generalize, given the many cultural and societal influences in different regions of the country and the diversity of health care in which people receive care.

Although the actual use of CAM therapies by people with PD is not known, research does offer clues to its acceptance and use. CAM use is growing in the PD community. A 2002 study noted that 40% and 54% of people with PD in the United States and United Kingdom, respectively, use CAM. A more recent analysis of six studies of PD CAM users reported a range from 25% to as high as 76%, with CAM use highest in Korea—which may reflect a great acceptance of healing and holistic therapies by Eastern cultures. Why individual patients choose CAM and the value they place on these therapies, then, is particularly relevant to their outcomes, both traditional and non-traditional. How this compares to the use, acceptance, and efficacy in people of Korean descent living in the United States or people of non-Korean descent is not known.

The most common therapies used by people with PD in the United States are vitamins, herbs, acupuncture, and massage. Use does not appear to correlate with disease duration or severity, but does correlate with younger age at onset, women, and education level.

Reasons for CAM use are varied but include factors such as the desire for control, distrust in health care, perceived safety, belief in "natural" products, fear of medicine side effects or toxicity, limited access to traditional treatment, cultural beliefs, marketing influences, and the belief in personal or innate healing.

There are some features specific to PD that peak interest in CAM therapies. One is the fear of pharmacological therapy. For example, a not uncommon misunderstanding is that levodopa, the therapeutic treatment "gold standard," is toxic to nerve cells or its efficacy is limited in years, therefore use should be delayed or even avoided. Although this is not true, I've found this misconception to be widespread and a strong driver of interest in more natural therapies. Another is the significant side effects associated with current PD medications. Finally, the burgeoning interest in exercise as not only a treatment arm of PD but as a focus and philosophy of care has led to the promotion of this positive lifestyle change as an important part of an individual's treatment plan.

Complementary and alternative therapies are not integrated into care. Only a fraction of people with PD inform their health care provider of CAM use. Estimates vary with anywhere from 10% to 50% of people with PD stating that they informed their health care provider of CAM use. It is not known why this information is not shared, although reasons could be many such as:

- Short appointment times
- Perceived clinician disinterest
- Lack of belief that these therapies have any impact on traditional therapy
- Concern about the clinician's negative judgment or lack of "belief" in these therapies
- Fear of ridicule

There is limited information and guidance when it comes to understanding the true benefits of these therapies and the costs and risks. Nine research trials designed to examine the effect of herbal therapies and medication use did not show a change in levodopa dose with these therapies, suggesting these therapies did not improve symptoms in a way that medication could be reduced.

Cost is not an insignificant factor given the added expense of these therapies on top of traditional medicines and the potential chronic use for lifelong conditions such as PD. Studies that analyze cost are few. The added cost of CAM therapies in Korea was US$102 compared to US$73 for traditional care. Patients seen in a neurology outpatient clinic in Europe spent 50 euros per month, even though, on average, they rated effect as "no improvement" or "some improvement."

It is clear that CAM use is increasing and of particular interest to people with PD. Chapter 3 explores how CAM therapies may work. Practical guidance is offered to help you make decisions about CAM, given that the scientific explanation for CAM's benefit and use is growing, even though much is still unknown or unexplained.

References
Medical Therapies

Miyaski, J. M. 2002. "Practice parameter: Initiation of treatment for Parkinson's disease: An evidence-based review: Report of the Quality Standards Subcommittee of the American Academy of Neurology." *Neurology* 8: 11–17.

Olanow, C. W., et al. 2009. "A double-blind, delayed-start trial of rasagiline in Parkinson's disease." *New England Journal of Medicine* 361: 1268–78.

Pahwa, R., et al. 2006. "Practice parameter: Treatment of Parkinson disease with motor fluctuations and dyskinesia (an evidence-based review): Report of the Quality Standards Subcommittee of the American Academy of Neurology." *Neurology* 66: 983–95.

Surgical Therapies

Farris, S., and M. Giroux. 2013. "Retrospective review of factors leading to dissatisfaction with subthalamic nucleus deep brain stimulation during long-term management." *Surgical Neurology International* 4: 69.

———. 2014. *DBS: A Patient Guide to Deep Brain Stimulation.* Englewood, CO: Movement & Neuroperformance Center Colorado.

Kahn, E. J. 2012. "Deep brain stimulation in early stage Parkinson's disease." *Neurology Neurosurgery Psychiatry* 83: 164–70.

Role of Integrative Medicine and Different Models of Care

Center for Mind-Body Medicine. www.cmbm.org

Chung, V., et al. 2006. "Efficacy and safety of herbal medicines for idiopathic Parkinson's disease: A systemic review." *Movement Disorders* 21: 1709–15.

Ferry, P., et al. 2002. "Use of complementary therapies and non-prescribed medication in patients with Parkinson's disease." *Postgraduate Medical Journal* 78: 612–14.

Ferry, P., M. Johnson, and P. Wallis. 2002. "Use of complementary therapies and non-prescribed medication in patients with Parkinson's disease." *Postgraduate Medical Journal* 78: 612–14.

Giroux, M. L., and S. Farris. 2008. "Treating Parkinson's disease: The impact of different care models on quality of life." *Topics in Geriatric Rehabilitation* 24: 83–89.

Grosset, D., et al. 2007. "A multicentre longitudinal observational study of changes in self-reported health status in people with Parkinson's disease left untreated at diagnosis." *Journal of Neurology, Neurosurgery, and Psychiatry* 78: 465–69.

Grosset, K. A., and D. G. Grosset. 2005. "Patient-perceived involvement and satisfaction in Parkinson's disease: Effect on therapy decisions and quality of life." *Movement Disorders* 20: 616–19.

Institute of Medicine. 2001. *Crossing the quality chasm: A new health system.* Washington, D.C.: National Academy Press.

Kim, S. R., et al. 2009. "Use of complementary and alternative medicine by Korean patients with Parkinson's disease." *Clinical Neurology and Neurosurgery* 111: 156–60.

Lorenc, A., et al. 2009. "How parents choose to use CAM: A systematic review of theoretical models." *BMC Complementary and Alternative Medicine.* 9: 8.

National Center for Complementary and Alternative Medicine. www.nccam.nih.gov.

Patient-Centered Outcomes Research Institute. www.pcori.org

Rajendran, P. R., R. E. Thompson, and S. G. Reich. 2001. "The use of alternative therapies by patients with Parkinson's disease." *Neurology* 11: 790–94.

Sackett, D. L., et al. 1992. "Evidence-based medicine: What it is and what it isn't. It's about integrating individual experience and the best external evidence." *British Medical Journal* 13: 71–72.

Wang, Y., et al. 2013. "Epidemiology of complementary and alternative medicine use in patients with Parkinson's disease." *Journal of Clinical Neuroscience* 20: 1065–67.

Zesiewicz, T., and M. L. Evatt. 2009. "Potential influences of complementary therapy on motor and non-motor complications in Parkinson's disease." *CNS Drugs* 23: 817–35.

CHAPTER
3

Scientific Evidence for a Holistic and Integrative Approach

Scientific evidence is often limited for integrative and healing therapies. It is often difficult to evaluate these treatments using the universally accepted controlled research trial. This type of research requires a tremendous amount of resources traditionally reserved to study traditional medical and surgical treatments and not community-based wellness and personal healing therapies. In addition, some therapies are simply too difficult to study in a controlled fashion. For instance, is it truly possible to create a placebo "treatment" for a study designed to test the effect of massage or meditation? Or what about therapies such as traditional Chinese medicine (TCM), which, by definition, use different combinations of herbal, nutritional, and healing therapies based on an individual's constitution and needs and, by definition, will vary from one person to the next?

These methods are designed to measure outcomes that are based on the assurance that all treatments, research environments, and research subjects are the same and treated the same to limit confounding variables that will influence results. These are limitations of current research methods when applied to integrative therapies. Many of the therapies described in this book, like TCM, are not standardized and the same integrative therapy will be delivered in a different way from one person to the next, and perhaps from one session to the next, as the therapy is tailored to the physical, spiritual, cultural, and emotional needs of that person.

The fact that research evaluating the effect of many integrative therapies is either limited or does not meet traditional rigorous methods leaves many patients and health care professionals skeptical of their value. This skepticism is enhanced by the fact that the mechanism by which these therapies work is often unknown. Furthermore, there is the reality that the business of personal wellness and supplement care is an aggressively marketed multibillion-dollar industry without the strict regulatory control applied to medicine and surgical therapies. For this reason it is important that you do your own research about risks and benefits and develop a true understanding of how a particular therapy or group of therapies would fit into your own healing regimen.

In this chapter, we discuss a few of the scientific principles pertinent to general health, personal healing, and brain function by which many of these therapies *can* work. The scientific evidence described in this section will give you a foundation by which you can analyze how a therapy can benefit you even when the specific action of a therapy is unknown or its use in Parkinson's disease (PD) is not tested. For instance, it is unknown how the energy therapy Reiki changes cellular physiology. But this therapy does engage the relaxation response, while also engaging the patient and practitioner in a therapeutic, supportive, and empathic relationship that in itself can bring a multitude of health benefits. Without a more specific scientific understanding of how Reiki therapy works, we can still apply these known mechanisms of action or beneficial factors to get results. In this case the decision to select Reiki can be made based on whether these values are important to you even when direct disease effect is unknown. Applying this strategy to your adaptation of a treatment will help you select or know that a therapy is worthwhile.

We begin with a review of the science behind the placebo, both as a reminder that this effect can be responsible for the outcomes of some therapies and is also an effect to be used to your advantage when possible. We will then review the physiology of the stress response, chemical influences on cellular healing, and the potential of neuroplasticity.

PLACEBO EFFECT AND ITS IMPORTANCE TO INTEGRATIVE MEDICINE

In medicine, the placebo effect is a measured change after an inactive treatment (sometimes referred to as a "sugar pill") is given to a person who otherwise "thinks" the treatment is real. The placebo is an important part of research designed to determine the true effect of a drug, surgery, or other treatment. Researchers can determine if a treatment is truly effective by comparing the differences measured between the placebo and treatment results.

Our emphasis is usually focused on positive effects. But negative effects can also occur. The *nocebo effect* is the term used to describe a negative response or outcome. The placebo is high in treatment studies for PD, sometimes accounting for up to 30% of a measured outcome or result in research studies. Supplements, medicines, acupuncture, fetal cell transplant, gene therapy, and deep brain stimulation (DBS) surgery are all associated with strong placebo effects in clinical studies. These observations are important for three reasons:

1. Some integrative therapies may be effective only due to their placebo effect.

2. The placebo can add to or subtract from the effect of a very specific and real treatment.

3. Knowledge of what influences the placebo response can be used to your advantage to improve the outcome of any treatment.

The role of the placebo is very important to integrative and holistic therapies especially since many of these therapies are not studied in ways to control for this effect. A positive or negative effect could simply be due to placebo and not the real treatment. In traditional medicine, research is designed to control for and subtract the placebo effect from the treatment effect to obtain the true effect of a treatment or surgery. The randomized placebo controlled research trial is designed with this intention. In a randomized trial, participants are randomly divided into two groups—one that gets the treatment under study or one that gets placebo "treatment" (e.g., sugar pill, sham surgery). Ideally, both research participants and the researcher are not aware of the group to which participants are assigned. This avoids any bias in measurement, observation, or interaction that researchers (or patients) can bring to the study that will influence results. In this way, the placebo group (i.e., results obtained from the group that unknowingly received inactive treatment) can be statistically compared to the active treatment group. If there is no difference between these two groups, the treatment is not considered effective even if benefits are measured. For example, the supplement coenzyme Q10 was associated with improved PD symptoms in an early small research study. However, similar findings were measured in the placebo group. As a result, researchers concluded that coenzyme Q10 (as given in the study) was not an effective PD treatment. Understanding that the placebo effect can explain why some therapies work for some people is an important first step in deciding if a therapy is right for you.

So What Causes the Placebo Effect, and How Can You Use It to Your Advantage?

Multiple psychological factors impact the strength of the placebo (or nocebo) effect. These factors include:

*   *Prior treatment experience or conditioned learning.* You will have a greater placebo effect with a treatment if you had a strong experience with a similar treatment in the past. In other words, each of us has past experiences, good and bad, and these experiences influence our future treatments. A positive experience will lead to a larger placebo effect and a negative experience

(side effect or no improvement) will lead to a larger nocebo effect. Psychologists call this response conditioned learning, since what we have learned from prior experiences *conditions* or influences our future experiences.

- *Expectations for treatment.* The placebo effect will change with the expectation attached to the treatment. If you believe or expect a treatment will have dramatic results, the placebo effect will be greater. If you believe a treatment will not work, then the nocebo effect will be stronger. This may be why studies show a greater placebo with a larger pill vs. smaller pill, brand name vs. generic medicine, invasive surgery vs. medicine, pill vs. injection, and yes, even natural therapy vs. prescription pill. An important example, commonly encountered in the clinic, is physical therapy. If you do not expect physical therapy to work, then the nocebo effect can actually "take away" from any potential benefits of this treatment.

- *Treatment value and meaning.* Placebo effect is influenced by the degree of value or personal meaning attached to a treatment. A treatment like stem cell, for instance, carries high hope and therefore high value. This could also apply to many integrative therapies, since many people place high value (and also high expectation) on natural or non-medical therapies, as these therapies align more closely with a personal philosophy or cultural belief related to natural health and healing. In this situation the placebo effect for the natural therapy would be even higher than a traditional therapy.

Personal experiences, expectations, ideals, and values contribute to the placebo effect and play an important role in integrative medicine. The following examples illustrate how these factors can influence treatment.

- *Side effects.* Many people have experienced side effects from prescription medicines. Indeed, more potent therapies sometimes have greater benefit and greater side effects. Some, but not all, natural therapies have lower side effect (but also less efficacy). The awareness that prescription drugs have side effects could in itself increase your risk of side effect from a future prescription medicine.

- *Health care delivery.* The U.S. health care experience is associated with increasing frustration and skepticism as medicine becomes institutionalized, technically advanced, financially and insurance driven, and depersonalized. Conversely, many integrative therapies are delivered in a quiet, empathic, and unrushed manner in a personalized environment that supports a sense of calm and relaxation. Medical doctors, hospitals, and clinics are associated with disease while spas, healing therapies, and vitamins are associated with wellness. It is likely that the experience, expectations, and values will change in these different environments. How and where the care is delivered, then, also changes your treatment outcome.

With even a superficial understanding of the placebo effect you can now appreciate the different impact that these scenarios will have on your treatment outcome.

What Is Known about the Placebo Effect and Parkinson's?

A placebo effect is measured in all studies of medicine. Even surgical results are influenced by the placebo effect. Fetal cells capable of producing dopamine were surgically implanted into the basal ganglia (requiring neurosurgery) of people with moderate stage PD. A sham surgery group (with patients taken to the operating room and prepared for surgery without the patients and researchers knowing if they did or did not receive surgery) was included to control for the placebo effect. The sham surgery group displayed improvement in both motor symptoms and dopamine PET scans[1] to a similar degree as the fetal cell group, leading the researchers to conclude that fetal cell was not an effective treatment. Gene therapy research has showed similar findings. Motor improvement in the group that received a gene designed to produce Neurturin, a growth factor capable of promoting nerve cell growth, did not differ statistically from the sham surgery group. Even DBS is influenced by the placebo effect. Patients with DBS do better after programming if they are coached by their programmer to expect positive results and will do poorly if given negative expectations.

The placebo effect may be particularly strong in PD due to the role of dopamine as part of the brain's reward system and the role of key frontal brain regions, which are part of the basal ganglia nerve circuitry affected by PD and are involved in thought patterns known to influence the placebo response.

Research studies prove that not only is the placebo effect significant in studies of PD treatment, but it is also associated with real biochemical and physiologic brain changes. For example, movement symptoms improve when PD individuals are unknowingly given a placebo (saline injection) instead of drug. What is remarkable is that individuals with the strongest placebo effect also have the greatest dopamine release in the basal ganglia as measured by brain PET scan. Further studies showed that this effect is also influenced by a person's prior experience with treatment (levodopa) and the individual's expectations or anticipation for therapeutic benefit.

How Does the Placebo Affect You?

The placebo effect is real and can cause positive or negative effects. When possible, choose therapies that have been studied in a controlled fashion over treatments that have only been studied using open label research (no placebo given and the entire group gets active treatment).

Not all treatments can or have been studied using the randomized placebo controlled trial. Just because a treatment has not been evaluated in this fashion does not mean it is ineffective. Some treatments just cannot be studied in this way and many alternative therapies fall into this category. For instance, it is difficult

---

[1] PET (positron emission tomography) scan is a nuclear medicine imaging scan that uses radioactive tracers to measure nerve cell activity and receptor and biochemical levels in the brain.

to find a placebo for treatments such as massage or acupuncture. That does not mean these treatments are not beneficial.

One must also be careful when choosing treatments that rely only on anecdotal reports and patient testimonies. Strong marketing techniques now widely accessible via the Internet are designed to sell and can be very persuasive. The following recommendations will help you find a treatment appropriate for you:

- If the treatment you are interested in is not yet proven effective, consider enrolling in a research trial if one is available. Research trials help to ensure safety, contribute to scientific knowledge, identify new treatments, and help advance care for all in the PD community.

- Talk to your health care provider about all treatments you are considering rather than "going it alone." Practical tips to guide this conversation are included in Part V, Personalize Your Care.

- Seek similar alternative treatments that are proven for other conditions in place of one not yet proven. An example may be the use of yoga, shown to be effective for other medical conditions, as compared to a new exercise fad.

- Consider the risk vs. benefit associated with any therapy or treatment. For instance, if you feel good after a massage and this treatment carries little risk to you (other than cost), then you may not need a higher level of proof of its direct effect. If a treatment carries higher risk, then it should require a greater level of proof as to benefit than a treatment with lower risk.

- Be cautious about therapies that claim to treat many conditions, promote cures, or achieve results that seem just too good to be true.

- Weigh the risk vs. benefit of treatment if there is high possibility that a treatment has a strong placebo effect. Be sure to include the cost of the treatment, and other treatments you will not be doing if you begin this treatment, as potential risks.

CLINICAL PEARL: HOW TO MAKE
THE PLACEBO WORK FOR YOU

Researchers spend time and effort to minimize the placebo response in experiments. As a person with PD, however, you are interested in the ultimate outcome: to feel better and reduce symptoms. You can enhance this outcome through the combined effect of real treatment and the placebo. This be done by matching your behavior to the factors that contribute to the placebo effect. Once again this very exercise reinforces the power of an integrative approach since it

(*continued*)

CLINICAL PEARL (*continued*)

highlights the real power of the mind and spirit in influencing how you feel. The following behaviors can help you harness your placebo effect.

- *Increase your level of expectation for therapy.* Understand the benefits and reinforce the positive.

- *Be aware of how your prior experience can affect current treatments.* Discuss your experience with your health care provider if you had a negative reaction to a treatment in the past. It is helpful to understand why you had a problem, ways that negative experiences can be circumvented going forth with new treatment, and how a new treatment is different. In this way you will be expecting a different response than that of your prior experience.

- *Actively participate.* A treatment has a greater chance of working if you are motivated to actively participate and work with your health care provider to make decisions for treatment. Aim to learn and understand what treatments can and cannot do and make a concerted effort to concentrate on the former and not the latter.

- *Include others in care.* Including your loved ones, family members, and friends in your decisions about care can help in many ways. The positive reinforcement and well-being you get from sharing, and the compassion, encouragement, and hope that are fostered as you begin your treatment, can go a long way toward successful outcomes.

- *Align with your beliefs.* Choose therapy that is in line with your values and beliefs. If you believe in the power of nutrition and supplements, ask your health care provider about treatments in this area. Use them along with, rather than in place of, the appropriate traditional therapy.

- *Combine treatments you believe in or that have special meaning to you with your traditional medical treatment.* For instance, it may be helpful to combine practices that are important to you to improve the benefit of a treatment. Examples include prayer, massage, meditation, and diet to aid the benefits of other treatment.

- *Reinforce positive learning.* Choose health care providers that you trust, actively listen to you, engage and educate you in

(*continued*)

CLINICAL PEARL (continued)

the decision making, and can demonstrate the benefits of a treatment.

- *Treat depression and anxiety.* These conditions affect your motivation, expectation, and perception that change can occur for the better.

- *Capitalize on the power of a good therapeutic relationship between you and your doctor or health care provider.* You are more apt to trust a provider who listens, understands, and is empathic and open to your needs, values, and ideas about your health care.

- *Optimize the setting of your care.* Start by preparing for your health care visits and arriving on time. This way you won't start your appointment stressed, rushed for time, or disappointed that you didn't get more out of your visit. The same is true for treatment you do at home. If exercise is prescribed, make it a positive experience: move the bicycle out of the basement, walk outside rather than on a treadmill, or choose a treatment like dance that is fun.

STRESS, HEALTH, AND ILLNESS

Your nervous system is constantly adapting and changing as it responds and reacts to your environment, activities, thoughts, and emotions. When dealing with a stressful situation, these nerve-driven changes help deal with and react to stress physically, emotionally, and cognitively. When stress is short-lived, these changes are necessary and adaptive. However, when stress is prolonged, these physiologic changes can threaten health.

The neurologic control of stress is a complex one involving specific regions of the brain and the autonomic nervous system. Key brain regions important to stress include the limbic system, hypothalamus, and frontal cortex. The limbic system is a specialized network or brain circuit that modulates our emotions, desires, and drives. The limbic system connects with higher-order brain centers involved in critical thinking, such as the frontal cortex, to place an additional layer of regulation over the more primitive limbic system to further influence how our thoughts, perceived threats, and emotions impact actions and behavior. The emotional brain and higher-order cognitive centers work together to guide the appropriate balance of activity, including activity of the hypothalamus and autonomic nervous system. The hypothalamus helps regulate our hormonal balance, circadian rhythms, sleep-wake cycle, temperature, and degree of alertness.

The hypothalamus in turn regulates brainstem and autonomic pathways called the parasympathetic and sympathetic nervous systems.

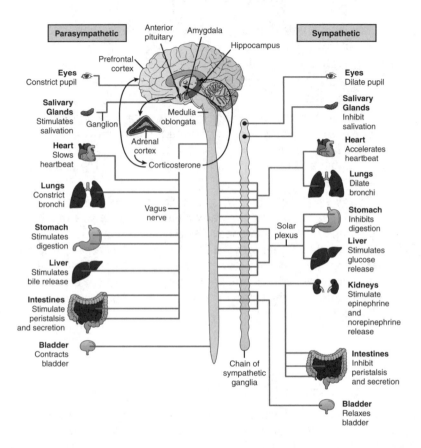

Every awake moment of every day is filled with a cascade of emotional, cognitive, and physical experiences that are registered by this complex network of neurons and that influence the neurologic output of these neurons. The meaning, benefits, or potential threat of a situation can serve as a control switch to preferentially engage and regulate how these interconnections control the autonomic nervous system.

The autonomic nervous system is divided into two branches designed to react and respond to the presence or absence of stress. These branches are defined by their triggers and effect. The key to health is a balance of these two systems:

1. The sympathetic nervous system engages the fight-or-flight response.
2. The parasympathetic nervous system engages the relaxation response.

The fight-or-flight or stress response is an adaptive response that allows the body to function at a heightened level of performance during a time of perceived threat or in high-intensity situations. A perceived threat could be something that would inflict physical, psychological, emotional, or personal harm. Body changes that occur when the sympathetic nervous system is activated include:

- Dilated pupils
- Sweating
- Rapid breathing
- Increased heart rate
- Increased blood pressure
- Increased alertness
- Increased muscle tension and shaking
- Activation of adrenal glands
- Shunting of blood from your internal organs to your muscles for action

The relaxation response balances the sympathetic system, allowing the body to return to a restorative and rejuvenated state once a perceived threat or a demanding or intense situation is over; this recovery brings readiness for the next threat. Body changes that occur when the parasympathetic nervous system is activated include:

- Decreased blood pressure
- Decreased pulse
- Deep, slow, rhythmic breathing
- Reduced anxiety
- Reduced muscle tension
- Improved mood
- Improved digestion
- Improved concentration
- Reduced pain threshold
- Shunting of blood to internal organs such as the gastrointestinal tract to aid digestion

This dual system of neurologic control works well for acute stress, allowing mind and body to take action during times of stress or threat and to rest once the threat or stressful event is over. The problem arises when we experience chronic stress. Chronic stress shifts the natural balance toward an overactive sympathetic response with fewer episodes of parasympathetic recovery.

Modern life brings many stressors: our busy jobs, traffic, unmet expectations, financial insecurities, multitasking, worries about the future, and even loneliness. Living with a chronic disease adds to this stress. If left unchecked, sympathetic nervous system overdrive leads to a sustained increase in stress hormones, especially one called cortisol. Chronic stress and elevated cortisol can cause anxiety, fatigue, depression, sleep problems, muscle pain (especially in the back, shoulder, and neck), weight problems, ulcers, high blood pressure, and heart disease. Other problems associated with chronic stress include decreased immune system function, reduced pain tolerance, increased risk of diabetes or heart disease, and even progression of illnesses such as cancer.

You are likely already aware of how stress changes your PD symptoms. Sometimes the first movement symptoms and the diagnosis of PD are noted during a time when life stress is particularly high. Stress can have immediate effects on symptoms, especially tremor, dyskinesia, and freezing of gait. Stress can also worsen other PD-related symptoms such as pain, dizziness, fatigue, sleep and mood disorders, cognitive difficulties, and hallucinations.

It is unknown if stress plays a direct role in the neurodegeneration seen with PD. Animal studies suggest that there is a connection. Exercise can protect dopamine nerve cells from damage caused by a neurotoxin, 1-methyl-4-phenyl-1,2,3,6-tetrahydropyridine (MPTP). If animals are subjected to stress, the protective effect of exercise is minimized. It is not known how this research applies to people, but the evidence to support the negative impact of stress on brain health is growing.

Chronic stress causes brain atrophy in crucial areas of the brain important for learning, movement, and emotional reasoning. Of interest, stress is shown to impact cellular DNA in ways that can lead to earlier cell death. Telomeres are protective caps at the ends of genes that influence cell health, aging, and even cell death. Increased cortisol levels found with chronic stress (or depression) are associated with reduced telomere length, indirectly connecting stress to cell death. A reduction in nerve growth factors needed to support nerve cell growth, an increase in inflammatory chemicals, and increased oxidative stress are additional ways that stress compromises brain cell function. Alterations in these important factors are also proposed mechanisms for nerve damage in PD, further strengthening the link between stress and disease.

Morning cortisol levels that increase with chronic stress are elevated in people with PD compared to age-matched individuals without the disease. The fact that medical treatment with levodopa reduces blood cortisol levels does suggest a relationship between low dopamine and chemical changes associated with stress as well as their reversal with treatment.

Fortunately, the impact of stress is reversible. Although you cannot remove all stress from your life, you can change how you react to stress. Relaxation techniques help you balance sympathetic and adrenal overdrive by increasing parasympathetic output and the relaxation response. You may notice that your PD symptoms feel better when you are relaxed, such as when you are enjoying a particular activity or are on vacation. This is the parasympathetic system at work! These changes are not limited to the autonomic nervous system: Brain imaging shows positive changes in the amygdala or brain distress center in people with PD after just eight weeks of stress-reducing, mindfulness-based therapy.

So How Do You Turn On and Maximize the Relaxation Response?

Mind-body therapies can effectively reduce the maladaptive neurologic changes associated with chronic stress. These simple techniques improve breathing, muscle tension, and mental calmness and focus attention in ways that enhance relaxation and bring out positive physiologic changes.

CELLULAR HEALING

PD is caused by cellular changes that ultimately lead to degeneration of nerve cells crucial for motor control. Genetics, exposure to environmental toxins, and cellular aging are factors that increase the risk of developing PD and offer strategies for prevention. Three cellular changes may cause or exacerbate PD-related cellular loss: mitochondrial dysfunction, oxidative stress, and cellular inflammation.

Mitochondrial Dysfunction

PD is associated with impaired brain cell mitochondrial function. The mitochondria are important structures located within cells that produce the needed energy for normal cell function and neurologic activity. Impaired energy production can have the effect of further increasing oxidative stress, altering calcium and electrolyte balance important for cell activity and genetically programmed cell survival vs. death, a process called apoptosis.

The discovery of the neurotoxin known as MPTP reinforces the causative role of mitochondria dysfunction and the powerful interplay between environment and cell health. In the early 1980s, scientists in California discovered a group of young individuals noted to have rapidly progressing parkinsonian symptoms. These individuals were exposed to MPTP, a lethal toxin sometimes produced as a by-product of illegally synthesized narcotics. What was soon discovered was that a breakdown product of MPTP selectively damages the same dopamine nerve cells involved in PD. MPTP is metabolized in the brain to a lethal chemical that is then taken up by nerve cells and blocks mitochondrial energy production. Certain pesticides, such as rotenone and paraquat, have since been discovered to have a similar effect. These findings further reinforce the link between environment, lifestyle, nerve cell health, and disease.

Oxidative Stress

Mitochondrial damage has many deleterious effects on nerve cell health, one of which is increased oxidative stress. Production of oxygen reactive free radicals is a chemical by-product of cellular metabolism. Oxidative stress occurs when production of these free radicals exceeds the cells buffering or neutralizing capacity. Free radicals are molecules that have one unpaired electron in their outer shell.

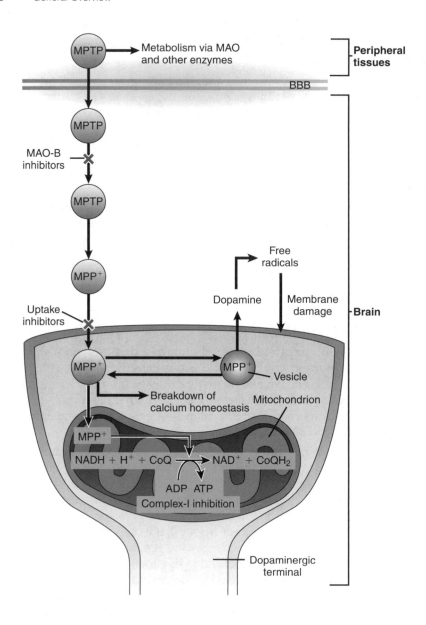

BBB = Blood-brain barrier
MPTP is converted to MPP$^+$ in the brain. MPP$^+$ interferes with mitochondrial
   energy production and dopamine to increase oxidative stress.

Unpaired electrons increase the chemical reactivity of molecules (molecules are
chemically stable when electrons are paired). In the body, oxygen is metabolized
to free radicals. These free radicals react with other molecules in the body, essentially stripping these molecules of electrons in an effort to produce a more stable
molecule. The resultant cascade of chemical reactions can lead to a domino effect

of cell damage if left unchecked. This process is called oxidative stress because the free radical cell damage is produced as a by-product of oxygen metabolism.

Dopamine nerve cells are especially vulnerable to oxidative stress since these nerve cells contain iron. Brain iron assists in the production of free radicals. Dopamine itself is metabolized in the brain through an oxidative process and the resulting metabolites further increase oxidative stress. Fortunately, your body has developed a defense system against this damage. Antioxidants are substances produced by the body or supplied by diet that can neutralize oxidative stress by donating electrons to the free radicals to make them stable. When abundant and working appropriately, these antioxidants mitigate damage of free radicals. When reduced, oxidative stress is free to inflict cell damage.

For example, glutathione, a powerful antioxidant, is reduced in aging and many chronic diseases. Brain levels are as much as 40% reduced in people with PD. It is conceivable that these changes play an important role in dopamine cell death.

Cellular Inflammation

Damaged nerve cells can cause inflammation and changes in immune cell reaction. Microglia are cells in the brain that coexist with nerve cells and support nerve cell health and function. Microglia are also important modulators of brain cell immune function. When activated these cells produce chemicals that produce inflammation called cytokines. In the case of MPTP-induced parkinsonism as described previously, MPTP cellular changes induce inflammation and this inflammation exists long after the toxin is removed.

Inflammation, then, may play a secondary role in disease causation and a primary one in progression. Indeed, epidemiological studies show that the chronic use of anti-inflammatory medicines such as pain medicines used to treat arthritis are associated with a reduced risk of PD.

Of interest, certain symptoms of PD may be more strongly associated with chronic inflammation. For instance, symptoms of depression, fatigue, and cognitive impairment are associated with higher levels of markers of cerebrospinal fluid inflammation as compared with PD individuals who do not have these problems. It remains to be determined whether anti-inflammatory strategies could selectively treat these symptoms.

How Do These Cellular Dysfunctions Offer Opportunity for You?

The influence of diet, lifestyle, and the environment on these potential causes of disease represent unique opportunities for treatment. For instance, antioxidants from foods, vitamins, and supplements can combat the oxidative cell damage associated with disease. Lifestyle factors such as exercise can reduce brain inflammation. Indeed, measures of inflammation are decreased after just eight weeks of moderate-intensity exercise (three one-hour sessions weekly). Even stress, the effects of which were reviewed earlier in this chapter, can play a critical role in disease. For instance, laboratory animals subjected to chronic stress exhibited a greater inflammatory response to a toxic brain injection, and this inflammatory response correlated with measures of movement difficulty and with dopamine nerve cell loss.

NEUROPROTECTION AND NEUROPLASTICITY

Neuroprotection

This is defined as the ability of a treatment to protect vulnerable neurons susceptible to cell damage or death in disease. In PD, a neuroprotective therapy would slow disease progression by reducing or delaying the degeneration of dopaminergic nerve cells. Animal models of PD offer a unique opportunity to study this hypothesis, and animal research to date suggests that exercise is neuroprotective. Neurotoxins capable of damaging dopamine neurons are injected into the basal ganglia of animals. The resulting dopamine nerve damage is associated with movement problems in these animals, similar to that seen in PD. This animal model represents a powerful laboratory tool to study the effect of potential treatments. Intensive exercise, often called forced exercise, reduces the degree of cell damage from the nerve toxin called 6-hydroxydopamine (6-OHDA) in rodents when started within 12 hours after injection. Fewer motor problems and an increase in nerve growth factors were associated with this effect. Similar studies showed a protective effect if animals were forced to exercise before being injected with this nerve toxin.

The evidence for exercise-induced neuroprotection in people with PD shows similar promise. A meta-analysis[2] of five studies researching the effect of exercise confirmed that exercise in early to mid-life reduces the risk of developing PD. Intense exercise improves motor symptoms, increases brain growth factors, and enhances dopamine activity when measured by PET scan. Most studies to date focus on high-intensity cardiac exercise such as bicycling or running, but whether other exercises also have this effect and how much exercise is needed to have these effects is unknown.

Neuroplasticity

Neuroplasticity encompasses neuroprotection, but includes broader changes in brain function in response to activity and experiences. Nerve cells have interconnections forming circuits that are part of even larger networks designed to work together. Neuroplasticity is defined as the ability of these interconnected brain cells to change or modulate connections and physiological processes with changes in activity. In essence, neuroplasticity allows the brain to respond, adapt, understand, and learn; it modulates brain activity or performance in response to the needs, changes, and challenges placed on us by our environment, activities, and experience.

---

[2] Meta-analysis is a statistical analysis of multiple studies in the attempt to identify similar trends and conclusions.

Neuroplasticity is a constant process that allows us to learn, adapt, and change. Neuroplasticity can be positive and adaptive or negative and maladaptive. For instance, exercise can have adaptive changes designed to strengthen sensorimotor, emotional, and cognitive networks, leading ultimately to better performance. Stressful environments, negative thoughts, hopelessness, or traumatic stress can produce changes in those regions of the brain that modulate distress and emotions (such as the amygdala described in the stress response), leading to symptoms such as depression, anxiety, or post-traumatic stress disorder (PTSD).

There are many examples of neuroplasticity resulting in improved brain function and performance. Low-impact exercise improves executive function, a type of cognitive change seen in PD. Exercise-induced improvement in mood and/or cognition is associated with brain growth factors and increased volume of the hippocampus, a brain region important in learning and memory. More expansive potential for neuroplasticity exists when selecting activities with sensorimotor integration and emotional, spiritual, or cognitive tasks. For examples of neuroplasticity in these domains, consider the following: Physical performance, cognitive ability, and emotional well-being can improve with meditation, and these results correlate with brain changes (both size and activity) measured in the frontal lobes and amygdala, the brain regions associated with high-level reasoning and distress, respectively. Not unexpected, exercise when performed outdoors has a greater impact on depression than exercise performed indoors. Finally, the simple act of holding the hand of a loved one during stress changes brain activity, suggesting that neuroplasticity may even be the reason why emotional connections and therapeutic touch are so important to healing and living with chronic disease.

In the right circumstance, then, our brains are developed to respond in ways that help us get the most out of activities that improve quality living. Consider adding positive neuroplasticity as a goal of therapy or treatment, whether it is the beneficial effect of medicine on the ability to move, a focused exercise plan, or exposure to emotionally positive events. As you review the information on lifestyle and integrative therapies, begin by choosing activities that are challenging and novel; require learning; are emotional and cognitively engaging; incorporate fun, music, or spirituality; and involve use of the senses in addition to movement.

CLINICAL PEARL: ENHANCE YOUR NEUROPLASTIC POTENTIAL

Neuroplasticity is about more than increasing your exercise intensity. There are many things you can do each day that engage and challenge and, in the process, promote positive brain change.

(*continued*)

CLINICAL PEARL (*continued*)

Take inventory of your day and think about how you might add activities for brain health based on these principles of neuroplasticity:

- *Learning.* Challenge your brain with activities that are new to you and require you to learn new things—innovative tasks, thoughts, or activities that require you to acquire new skills or ideas, such as dancing, singing, acting, painting, or playing an instrument.

- *Complexity.* More challenging activities require you to focus and may take practice to perform. For example, you might consider substituting a workout on the weight machine or the treadmill with a performance task that requires attention and practice and that challenges you, such as yoga or non-contact boxing, Feldenkrais Method®, dance, or rock climbing.

- *Practice and intensity.* Practice makes perfect and effort gets results. Neuroconnections in specific brain circuits associated with a particular activity will strengthen the more you perform that activity. Think about your performance when putting forth effort. The goal is not to do more, but to do the activity with a focus on performance. For example, walking faster and longer will improve cardiac output and nerve function, but more is not always better as you can reinforce poor biomechanics. Walking faster while paying attention to posture, arm swing, and stride length will strengthen nerve connections associated with improving your gait.

- *Choosing positivity.* You will find that certain activities enhance positive feelings or attitude and a sense of possibility and control. Workshops, classes, and group activities not only add encouragement and keep you motivated, but the positive support and social interactions that make you feel good about your experience will lead to changes in emotional control areas of the brain such as the limbic system.

- *Adding meaning.* Some activities bring a sense of personal meaning, significance, or spiritual growth. Is there an opportunity to volunteer or teach and connect with others in a meaningful way? The impact of meaning and the quality of your experience is also significant as is highlighted through observations. For example, the impact of exercise differs depending on whether it is performed in a group, is an activity you enjoy, or is experienced in nature rather than indoors.

(*continued*)

CLINICAL PEARL (*continued*)

- *Being present.* Mindfulness means being present in the moment. Don't just go through the motions but expand your experience and the results of your activity by adding awareness of your senses, thoughts, emotions, body movement, and other sensations.

- *Integration.* Brain activity is not limited to individual circuits working in isolation but also involves an integration of brain regions and circuits. Enhance neuroconnections throughout the brain by choosing activities that integrate your senses, motion, emotions, and spirit. For instance, music, dance, and music therapy effectively tap into each of these areas while adding challenge and fun. In the case of moving to music, difficult movements also become easier since our brains are "hardwired" to move to the beat.

PRACTICAL CONSIDERATIONS

Just because there is limited research on the use, benefits, safety, and cost of complementary and alternative medicine (CAM) therapies does not mean these therapies are ineffective. Adopting a practical approach in regard to a theoretical basis for use, therapist selection, integration, and cost will guide your selection of the best therapies and help keep you safe.

As you read through this book you will likely ask this question: What is the best therapy for me? There is no right or wrong answer, since the benefits of specific CAM therapies depend on many factors, including whether they align with your belief and value system, are therapies you enjoy and that give you a sense of relief or well-being, and are safe, affordable, and therefore sustainable. Just as each person's medications are tailored to his or her needs, so are integrative therapies. In the following chapters we will review how these therapies may work in order to help you decide if a therapy is right for you.

Other Considerations Affecting Choice

Think about what is going well in your life, what is missing, and what you enjoy. Remember the concept of life in balance and moderation. You might consider setting priorities based on this concept. Is your exercise level appropriate? What about your diet, level of stress, and your supportive relationships or spiritual self? Do you have opportunities to relax? Do you need extra guidance from a coach or therapist? Do you do better in a group or in one-on-one activities, with individual or self-guided care? Worksheets to help you with these questions and similar questions designed to *personalize* your program are available in the last chapter of this book.

Safety

Some of the treatments and therapies that you will learn about in later chapters have strong scientific evidence to support their use in PD. Others are just beginning to be studied but have proven benefits in other diseases or symptoms. Yet many more have little, if any, scientific evidence for benefit and rely instead on anecdotal reports and individual stories claiming benefits big and small.

As mentioned previously, it does not necessarily mean that a treatment is ineffective if scientific evidence is lacking for a specific treatment. It may be that studies simply have not been done or are difficult to perform in a vigorous controlled trial and therefore do not meet the rigorous standards set forth by traditional evidence-based medicine. For instance, you learned about the value of the randomized controlled research study when we reviewed the placebo effect. Yet some therapies simply cannot be tested in this manner. Massage therapy, for instance, is very difficult to study in this manner. Supplements, on the other hand, are easier to study in this manner. Therefore, it is important to look for results from randomized controlled research trials for any supplement before taking.

Alternatively, just because individual stories or marketing materials claim that a treatment works does not mean that it does indeed work. Once again the power of placebo—driven by perceived value, expectations, and prior experiences—can be at play. Many people place great value and have high expectations for certain therapies. For many of you reading this book, this may be especially true for treatments thought of as *natural* or *holistic*.

How can you navigate these murky waters given all of this uncertainty? One way is to analyze all treatments on a risk vs. benefit scale. If risk of a treatment is low, then perhaps you can accept less scientific vigor for this treatment. Conversely, if risk of a treatment is documented, this risk must be weighed against benefit. In this situation, greater evidence of benefit is important given greater risk. Risk comes in many forms, including cost and what you are *not* doing because of the treatment. Take the example of massage therapy. The risk may be small; however, this risk can increase considerably if the financial cost is so high that you cannot afford to eat right. Risk is also high if massage is used in place of effective treatments such as physical therapy designed to target and combat muscle and joint rigidity, weakness, and problems of posture and biomechanics.

The Food and Drug Administration (FDA) regulates medical and surgical therapies to ensure the highest possible public safety and efficacy. Medical clinicians must complete formal education, training, and competency certification. This is not true for many non-traditional therapists or healing specialists. Do your research. Are specific training programs or certifications available in the field? If so, is a practitioner you are interested in certified or appropriately trained? How many years of experience do practitioners have, and what is their knowledge of PD?

Are they making extravagant claims that are almost too good to believe, or do they offer therapy that is directed by goals, with criteria to follow when treatment is not working? Use the Practitioner Checklist (found in Part V of this book) to help you select a practitioner.

Finally don't forget to talk to your health care provider about your interest in adding these therapies to your treatment regimen. This is a very important step if you are to truly integrate and optimize these treatments and minimize risk. You may find that your physician or health care provider is skeptical and may even be resistant to your desire to include non-traditional therapies, due to lack of evidence and understanding of the treatment. If this is the case, we offer the following tips to help you during a discussion with your provider. (You can also refer to the Physician Discussion Tool, found in Part V.)

CLINICAL PEARL: HOW TO TALK TO YOUR NEUROLOGIST ABOUT INTEGRATIVE THERAPIES

The following helpful tips, with illustrative examples of what to say, can help you when talking to your doctors, even if they are skeptical of integrative therapies.

- Begin with a discussion of your goal for treatment before moving on to discussion of a specific treatment. For example: "I am interested in finding non-medical ways of helping my back pain. My goal is to improve pain so that I can reduce reliance on pain medicine."

- Reinforce your self-care values and priorities: "I have always been interested in personal healing and believe that certain non-traditional therapies can be helpful. Trying these therapies also gives me a sense of hope and control, which is important to me."

- Describe the mechanism (with the help of this book) by which you believe a certain therapy may help. For example: "Research supports the use of acupuncture for pain."

- Reinforce the fact that you would like to begin this therapy for your own self-care and not to replace appropriate traditional therapies your doctors may prescribe: "I know this is not the only solution, so I will continue to take my medicines and see the physical therapist prescribed to help my back."

(continued)

CLINICAL PEARL (*continued*)

● Discuss the potential risk of the treatment and what you will measure as a sign of both progress and a reason to continue, limit, or stop treatment. For example: "According to my research, the risk of acupuncture is low. I will be sure to find an acupuncturist who has the certification and training necessary. There is cost associated with this treatment, so I will discuss my pain control goals with the therapist before starting and agree on a specific number of treatments, and then reevaluate the benefit. I will also be sure not to change any medicines without discussing with you [my neurologist] first."

References
Placebo Effect and Its Importance to Integrative Medicine

Ceregene Inc. "News in Context: Second Phase 2 trial CERE-120 yields disappointing results." April, 19 2013. www.michaeljfox.com

Frenkel, O. 2008. "A Phenomenology of the 'placebo effect': Taking meaning from the mind to the body." *Journal of Medicine and Philosophy* 33: 58–79.

Lindston, S. C., et al. 2010. "Effects of expectation on placebo-induced dopamine release in Parkinson disease." *Archives General Psychiatry* 67: 857–65.

Mercado, R., et al. 2006. "Expectation and placebo effect in patients with subthalamic nucleus deep brain stimulation." *Movement Disorders* 21: 1457–61.

Thompson, W. G. 2005. *The Placebo Effect and Health: Combining Science and Compassionate Care.* Amherst, NY: Prometheus Books.

Stress, Health, and Illness

Epel, E., J. Daubenmier, and J. Muskowitz, et al. 2009. "Can meditation slow rate of cellular aging? Cognitive stress, mindfulness, and telomeres." *Annals of the New York Academy of Science* 1172: 34–53.

Hemmerle, A., J. Herman, and K. Seroogy. 2012. "Stress, depression, and Parkinson's disease." *Experimental Neurology* 233: 79–86.

Howells, F., V. Russell, M. Mabandla, and L. Kellaway. 2006. "Stress reduces the neuroprotective effect of exercise in an animal model of Parkinson's disease." *Behavioral Brain Research* 165: 210–20.

Muller, T., and S. Muhlack. 2007. "Acute levodopa intake and associated cortisol decrease in patients with Parkinson's disease." *Clinical Neuropharmacology* 30: 101–6.

Pickut, B. A., et al. 2013. "Mindfulness-based intervention in Parkinson's disease leads to structural changes on MRI: A randomized controlled trial." *Clinical Neurology Neurosurgery* 115: 2419–25.

Skogar, O. 2011. "Diurnal salivary cortisol concentrations in Parkinson's disease: increased total secretion and morning cortisol concentrations." *International Journal of General Medicine* 4: 561–69.

Cellular Healing

De Pablos, R. M., et al. 2014. "Chronic stress enhances microglia activation and exacerbates death of nigral dopaminergic neurons under conditions of inflammation." *Neuroinflammation* 24: 11–34.

Hall, L. D., et al. 2013. "Cerebrospinal fluid inflammatory markers in Parkinson's disease." *Brain, Behavior, and Immunity* 33: 183–89.

Henchcliffe, C., and M. F. Beal. 2008. "Mitochondrial biology and oxidative stress in Parkinson's disease pathogenesis." *Nature Clinical Practice Neurology* 4: 600–9.

Hwang, O. 2013. "Role of oxidative stress in Parkinson's disease." *Experimental Neurobiology* 22: 11–17.

Langston, J. W., and J. Palfreman. 2104. *The Case of the Frozen Addicts*. Amsterdam: IOS Press.

Sian, J., et al. 1994. "Alterations in glutathione levels in Parkinson's disease and other neurodegenerative disorders affecting basal ganglia." *Annals of Neurology* 36: 348–55.

———. 1999. "MPTP induced Parkinsonism." In *Basic Neurochemistry: Molecular, Cellular, and Medical Aspects* 6th ed., edited by G. J. Siegel et al. Philadelphia: Lippincott-Raven. www.ncbi.nlm.gov/books/NBK27974/

Zoldz, J. A., et al. 2014. "Moderate-intensity interval training increases serum brain-derived neurotrophic factor level and decreases inflammation in Parkinson's disease patients." *Journal of Physiology and Pharmacology* 65: 441–48.

Neuroprotection and Neuroplasticity

Beal, E. B., et al. 2013. "The effect of forced-exercise therapy for Parkinson's disease on motor cortex functional connectivity." *Brain Connect* 3: 190–98.

Coan, J. A., et al. 2006. "Lending a hand: Social regulation of the neural response to threat." *Psychology Science* 17: 1032–39.

Farley, B. G., et al. 2008. "Intensive amplitude-specific therapeutic approaches for Parkinson's disease: Toward a neuroplasticity-principled rehabilitation model." *Topics in Geriatric Rehabilitation* 24: 99–114.

Fraxzitta, G., et al. 2014. "Intensive rehabilitation increases BDNF serum levels in parkinsonian patients: A randomized study." *Neurorehabilitation and Neural Repair* 28: 163–68.

Hannan, A. J. 2014. "Environmental enrichment and brain repair: harnessing the therapeutic effects of cognitive stimulation and physical activity to enhance experience-dependent plasticity." *Neuropathology and Applied Neurobiology* 40: 13–25.

Hirsch, M. A., and B. G. Farley. 2009. "Exercise and neuroplasticity in persons living with Parkinson's disease." *European Journal of Physical and Rehabilitative Medicine* 45: 215–29.

Lazar, S. W., et al. 2005. "Meditation experience is associated with increased cortical thickness." *Neuroreport* 16: 1893–97.

Naoki, T., et al. 2010. "Exercise exerts neuroprotective effects on Parkinson's disease model of rats." *Brain Research* 1310: 200–7.

Petzinger, G. M., et al. 2013. "Exercise-enhanced neuroplasticity targeting motor and cognitive circuitry in Parkinson's disease." *Lancet Neurology* 12: 716–26.

Xu, Q., et al. 2010. "Physical activities and future risk of Parkinson disease." *Neurology* 75: 341–48.

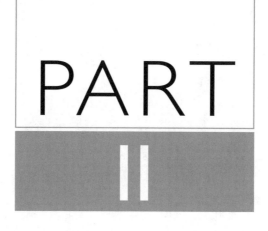

PART

II

General Health and Lifestyle Medicine

You will not feel your best if you focus your treatment and energy solely on your Parkinson's disease (PD). Fortunately, treatment and lifestyle choices important for general health are also important for PD. In this section, we focus on healthy aging, medical problems more common in PD, and lifestyle choices that are so important to living your best.

CHAPTER

4

Healthy Aging

Simple and practical lifestyle changes are perhaps the best place to start, whether you are living with Parkinson's disease (PD), have a loved one with PD, or are simply interested in feeling better and warding off disease. With this focus you gain a lifetime of positive health effects and the added benefit of a sense of control so often lost when living with a chronic condition.

PD is a progressive disease with an average age of onset just under 60 years. As medicine becomes increasingly specialized, the focus of treatment and self-care all too often becomes limited to the disease itself and not the other contributing health factors that lead to well-being and improved function. Living well with PD also means aging well. The science of aging is a burgeoning field whose scope is broader than that covered in this book. What is included on this topic is a review of the conditions that have increased occurrence with aging and, if present, will impact how you will feel and function with PD. The topics chosen for inclusion in this section are based on the most common general health questions and concerns discussed with my patients in the clinic.

- Cardiac health
- Stroke prevention
- Dementia and cognitive health

- Balance and walking
- Gastrointestinal (GI) health
- Skin, bone, and dental health

CARDIAC HEALTH

Heart disease is the number-one cause of mortality for aging adults, accounting for over 40% of all deaths. Heart failure is 2.27 times greater in people with PD than those without. Despite this fact, there is little emphasis on a heart-healthy lifestyle and treatment in PD clinics. Long-term symptoms and/or associated problems of heart disease important to people with PD include:

- Shortness of breath
- Exercise intolerance and decreased stamina
- Fatigue
- Stroke
- Cognitive impairment
- Depression

Prevention of heart disease and even reversal of atherosclerotic plaque in blood vessels are possible. Certain risk factors for heart disease cannot be changed, such as family history and gender (although men are at greater risk than women, risk in postmenopausal women approaches that of men). Fortunately, the majority of risk factors are modifiable.

Medical factors that increase the risk of heart disease include:

- Hypertension
- Diabetes
- High cholesterol
- Depression
- Sleep apnea
- Oral/gum disease
- Use of certain types of non-steroidal anti-inflammatory medicines (NSAIDs)
- Elevated homocysteine

Lifestyle risk factors associated with heart disease are:

- Smoking
- Alcohol abuse
- Sedentary lifestyle
- Stress
- Obesity, especially when associated with increased waist circumference (waistline)

Lifestyle changes that can *reduce* your risk of heart disease include:

- Aerobic and resistance training
- Stress management
- Diet (with the Mediterranean and DASH diets in particular; both are reviewed in Chapter 5)

These findings are based on many research studies, the most comprehensive of which is the Framingham Heart Study. The Framingham Heart Study began in 1948 and was designed to identify the risk factors for heart disease by examining a group of men and women every two years. Medical history, physical examination, and lifestyle factors were analyzed from 5,209 people in the original group from Framingham, Massachusetts; a second generation of 5,124 individuals in 1974; and now a third generation of study participants enrolled in 2002. Results of this study led to the Framingham Heart Disease Risk Score, a simple tool used to calculate the 10-year risk of developing heart disease. This tool uses information such as age, gender, cholesterol level, presence of hypertension, and smoking history to estimate risk. Framingham Risk Calculators[1] are available online to determine your risk.

Certain cardiac (and stroke) risk factors deserve special attention as they relate to PD. Sleep apnea and depression are PD non-motor symptoms that also increase cardiac and stroke risk. Diabetes increases risk of heart disease and appears to be more common in PD. The association of cholesterol and PD is confusing, with high levels of cholesterol showing an increased risk in some studies and reduced risk in others. Low cholesterol levels are also reported to be associated with increased risk, yet statin medicines used to treat and lower cholesterol may reduce risk. Given this complex maze, cholesterol should be treated if high and very low levels should be avoided. Finally, elevated homocysteine increases risk of blood clotting, stroke, and heart disease. Levodopa increases homocysteine levels. (Chapter 6 illustrates the complex relationship among homocysteine, B vitamins, and levodopa.)

STROKE PREVENTION

Stroke is the number-four cause of death in adults. Whether the risk of stroke is different in PD is not clear, with research findings showing no difference, a reduced risk, or increased risk based on the study analyzed. Lower risk of stroke in one study was thought to be related to the observation that fewer people with PD smoke. A more recent study of 820 people with PD found that stroke was increased by a factor of three to four, compared with the general population—a risk that was further increased by high lipid levels, diabetes, and high doses of levodopa.

---

[1] Framingham Risk Calculators for various conditions are available at www.framingham heartstudy.org/risk-functions.

The connection between levodopa and stroke may be related to the impact of this medicine on blood levels of the amino acid homocysteine. Homocysteine is elevated by levodopa metabolism. High levels of homocysteine may be toxic to nerve cells by elevating oxidative stress and inflammation. Homocysteine is also associated with increased blood clotting that can lead to stroke or coronary artery blockage (heart attack). Despite these associations there is no evidence to date that shows that lowering homocysteine levels reduces the risk of dementia, stroke, or heart disease.

Stroke symptoms can impact movement and balance through loss of sensation, impaired vision, or muscle weakness. Stroke symptoms that are important to people with PD include:

- Muscle weakness
- Speech and swallowing problems
- Balance and walking problems
- Visual disturbances
- Sensory disturbances
- Depression
- Cognitive impairment

Stroke can also cause a condition called vascular parkinsonism, further highlighting the importance of brain vascular health. Vascular parkinsonism, sometimes called lower body parkinsonism, is associated with postural instability, shuffling gait, and dementia.

Stroke risk factors and prevention are similar to those listed for prevention of heart disease. Blood clotting disorders, heart failure, and atrial fibrillation are additional factors that can increase stroke risk.

DEMENTIA AND COGNITIVE HEALTH

Dementia is a decline in thinking abilities significant enough to impact daily life. It is estimated that up to 30% of people with PD will develop dementia. The risk of dementia increases with age and the severity of motor symptoms. Dementia in PD could be related to the disease or causes such as vascular dementia and/or Alzheimer's disease. Risk factors and preventive strategies for dementia are similar to that for stroke and heart disease. Additional risk factors for dementia include:

- Age
- Apo lipoprotein e4 gene (APOE)[2]

---

[2] The APOE gene produces the protein Apo lipoprotein E, which combines with fats in the body to form lipoproteins important to fat and cholesterol distribution in the body.

- Head trauma
- High blood pressure
- Diabetes
- High cholesterol
- Cardiac disease and brain vascular disease
- Lower level of education
- Limited emotional support
- Limited creative, social, and cognitive engagement

Of interest is the inclusion of social and personal experiences such as the absence of support, low level of formal education, and limited level of life engagement as these experiences or behaviors are also important contributors to neuroplasticity, as discussed in Chapter 3.

BALANCE AND WALKING

Problems with walking, balance, and falls increase with age, but is this an inevitable part of aging? It is interesting to note that walking speed predicts longevity in older adults. Scientific studies note decreased walking speed, stride length, and postural sway with aging. Decreased walking speed and stride length may be a compensation for flexed posture, lack of flexibility, and balance problems. Cognitive problems that will change walking with age include problems with multitasking, attention, and speed of cognitive processing. Visual problems, arthritis, joint replacement, and peripheral neuropathy can dramatically impact gait. Even the fear of falling can increase falls.

Peripheral neuropathy deserves special mention since as many as 8% of older adults exhibit this problem. Peripheral neuropathy is associated with a loss of sensation beginning in the feet, progressing up the legs, and even involving the hands in severe cases. Symptoms if present are described as numbness, tingling, or burning sensation. Peripheral neuropathy has many medical causes, but the most common are diabetes, thyroid disease, vitamin B12 deficiency, and blood protein disorders. Diabetes is more common in PD. Studies controlling for diabetes and other factors suggest that peripheral neuropathy may also be higher in PD. Possible causes include a deficiency in vitamin B12 caused by levodopa-induced elevation in homocysteine levels.

Walking and balance require the neurologic integration of multiple nerve pathways and the precise control of joint, posture, and body mechanics. Primary neurologic systems that impact gait include vision, skin and joint position sensation, and vestibular control. These systems work together to control center of gravity, muscular and skeletal control of movement, movement velocity, control of postural sway, and reaction to change in stimulus or environment. These neurologic systems are depicted in the following figure.

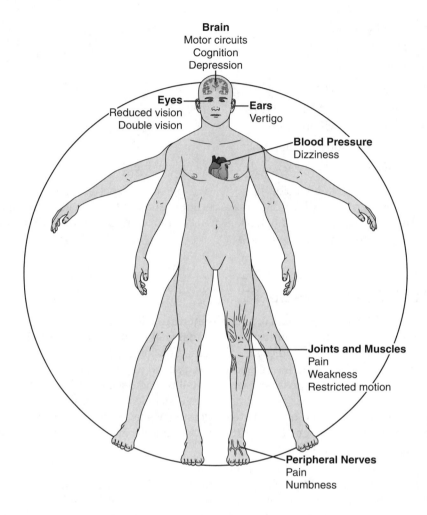

Brain
Motor circuits
Cognition
Depression

Eyes
Reduced vision
Double vision

Ears
Vertigo

Blood Pressure
Dizziness

Joints and Muscles
Pain
Weakness
Restricted motion

Peripheral Nerves
Pain
Numbness

Common age-related medical conditions and risk factors (not including brain and spinal cord disease) for walking and balance problems include:

- Vision loss, such as cataracts, glaucoma, or macular degeneration
- Vestibular or "inner ear" problems
- Cognitive decline
- Depression
- Low blood pressure
- Peripheral neuropathy
- Pain
- Spinal stenosis, joint disease, and joint replacement
- Muscle weakness

- Vitamin E, D, B12, and thyroid deficiencies
- Cardiopulmonary disease
- Malnutrition
- Alcoholism

GI HEALTH

PD-related and aging-related GI problems range from difficulty swallowing and pooling of saliva to gastric bloating and reflux, delayed stomach emptying, and slow movement of digested food through the intestinal tract. Levodopa absorption could be impaired if delayed gastric emptying and constipation are problems since this medicine must reach the small intestine for absorption.

The following chart illustrates the important relationship among your diet, lifestyle, and GI health.

SYMPTOM	IMPROVES	WORSENS
Swallowing	Foods with soft consistency	Water/thin liquids Dry foods
Gastric reflux, bloating, and delayed emptying	Small, more frequent meals Ginger	Diet high in fats Obesity, especially abdominal fat
Constipation	Fluids Fiber Probiotics	Anticholinergic medicines, amantadine Inactivity Dehydration

Gastric and duodenal ulcers are common in PD. *Helicobacter pylori* (*H. pylori*) is a bacteria present at higher levels in the gastric acid of individuals with ulcers and people with PD. *H. pylori* may also increase stroke and dementia risk through a combination of infection-induced inflammatory and immune reactions. Recent evidence suggests that treating and eliminating *H. pylori* may enhance the absorption of levodopa.

The GI tract has many roles, from digestion of food and absorption of nutrients and medicines into the bloodstream, to processing vitamins, breaking down fats, and removing toxins. Pathological findings showing the earliest evidence of PD nerve damage in the intestinal tract suggest that the GI tract is a portal for neurotoxin exposure and entry into the body. The intestines is anatomically linked to the brain by a nerve called the vagus nerve. This nerve may provide a pathway for neurochemical changes to gain entrance in the brain.

Gut bacteria and environmental toxins could work together to produce inflammation, oxidative stress, and leaky gut (inflammation of the bowel lining, causing increased permeability or leakage of damaging chemicals and bacterial products into the bloodstream). A small study of nine people with PD identified increased GI "leakiness," which correlated with bacterial toxin products that cause inflammation.

Reduced GI motility in PD could encourage bacterial overgrowth and the changes described. Treatment could focus on improved intestinal transit and dietary change as follows:

- Increase your intake of fluids, especially water.
- Limit sugary foods such as high fructose corn syrup and processed foods.
- Increase dietary fiber to 20 to 30 grams daily.
- Add probiotics to help restore beneficial bowel bacteria and treat symptoms of constipation.

SKIN, BONE, AND DENTAL HEALTH

Melanoma

The risk of skin cancer increases with age and with PD. Melanoma is a potentially fatal form of skin cancer. After examining over 2,000 people with PD, researchers conclude that the risk of developing melanoma is 2.24 times than the general population. Skin examinations by your general doctor or dermatologist are strongly advised since melanoma is life-threatening if found late, but treatable if diagnosed early. Report any change in mole size or appearance (irregularity, bleeding, or pigmentation) to your health care provider.

Overexposure to ultraviolet rays from sunshine or tanning beds can increase skin cancer risk. Exposure to sunshine between the hours of 10 a.m. and 4 p.m. is particularly harmful due to high levels of ultraviolet radiation during these times. The Centers for Disease Control and Prevention (CDC) recommend avoiding sun exposure during these times, using sunscreen, wearing sunglasses and protective clothing, and avoiding indoor tanning beds to reduce your risk of skin cancer. This approach to minimizing the risk of sun exposure may also keep you from getting the benefits of sunshine—namely, vitamin D.

Bone Health

Strong associations exist between PD health and vitamin D, otherwise known as the *sunshine vitamin*. Vitamin D is produced via skin exposure to ultraviolet rays from the sun. No one knows how much sun exposure is safe and many variables such as skin color, ethnicity, geography, and time of day will be factors. Lower levels of vitamin D are noted early in diagnosis and when depression and cognitive problems are present. Low levels of vitamin D, particularly below 30 nmol/L, also compromise bone health since vitamin D is involved in calcium and bone metabolism.

Vitamin D increases calcium absorption through the intestines and into bone. Strong bones reduce the risk of bone fracture from falls and are important for good posture. Bone mass is at its peak in our mid-30s and declines thereafter.

Osteopenia and osteoporosis ("porous bones") are the terms used for mild and more severe loss of bone density and strength, respectively. Symptoms of osteoporosis are bone pain, loss of height with stooped posture, and fractures, most common in the hips, spine, or wrist. When osteoporosis is severe, fractures can occur even after simple tasks that put strain on your skeletal system, such as leaning over to pick up a heavy object.

Bone loss increases after menopause when estrogen declines in women and continues to decline with age. Although women are at greater risk, men over the age of 75 and with low testosterone levels are also at risk. Other factors that increase your risk of osteoporosis include alcoholism, smoking, and ingestion of soda, aluminum-containing antacids, and corticosteroid medicines. The following list highlights additional risk factors for osteoporosis in PD:

- Low vitamin D levels
- Low calcium intake, which can be due to poor diet, interference with medicines, or reduced absorption because of GI disorders
- Lack of sun exposure, especially if movement problems keep you indoors
- Limited weight-bearing exercise, which is important for bone remodeling
- Thin body habitus or body size
- Depression, although how this is a risk is not known. One study showed people on selective serotonin reuptake inhibitors (SSRI) antidepressants were at risk. The risk could be related to other factors, such as changes in diet and physical activity with depression

There are many things you can do to improve your bone health and prevent bone loss:

- *Exercise.* Just like muscles, bones are stronger when used to bear weight. Jumping, walking, stair climbing, and dancing are examples of weight-bearing exercise.
- *Talk to your health care provider about screening tests.* Radiology tests can measure bone density to identify if you are at risk or have osteoporosis or osteopenia. Ask your doctor about screening with a DEXA or dual-energy x-ray absorptiometry scan if you are over age 65 or if you have any risk factors.
- *Get your vitamin D level checked.* Your health care provider can check your level by ordering a simple blood test.
- *Obtain adequate amounts of calcium and vitamin D in your diet.* More information on foods fortified with calcium and vitamin D is included in Part III: Integrative Therapies.
- *Get outdoors!*

Dental Health

Oral and dental health and care is often overlooked when it comes to health and disease. Difficulty chewing or brushing, ill-fitting dentures, and dry mouth from medications can cause dental problems in PD. Gingival and periodontal disease (gum disease) increases oral bacteria, which increases inflammation and inflammatory markers and in turn increases risk of heart disease. Poor oral health and bacteria also increase the risk of pneumonia due to aspiration of saliva in more advanced disease. The following tips can improve your oral health:

- Ask your dentist for a mouthwash designed to treat gingival plaque.
- Drink plenty of fluids.
- Use an electric toothbrush if brushing is difficult due to tremor of other symptoms.

References

Cardiac Health

Doherty, G. H. 2013. "Homocysteine and Parkinson's disease: A complex relationship." *Journal of Neurological Disorders* 1: 107.

Driver, J. A. 2008. "Prospective cohort study of type 2 diabetes and the risk of Parkinson's disease." *Diabetes Care* 31: 2003–5.

Eckel, R. G., et al. 2014. "2013 AHA/ACC guideline on lifestyle management to reduce cardiovascular risk: A report of the American College of Cardiology, American Heart Association Task Force on Practice Guidelines." *Journal of the American College of Cardiology* 63: 2960–84.

Framingham Heart Risk Calculator. http://cvdrisk.nhlbi.nih.gov/

Hu, G. 2010. "Total cholesterol and the risk of Parkinson's disease: A review for some new finding." *Parkinson's Disease* Article ID 836962.

Huang, X., et al. 2014. "Serum cholesterol, statin, and Parkinson's risk in the Atherosclerosis Risk in Communities (ARIC) study. *Neurology* 82: S17.006

Zesiewicz, T. A., et al. 2004. "Heart failure in Parkinson's disease: analysis of the United States Medicare current beneficiary survey." *Parkinsonism and Related Disorders* 10: 417–20.

Stroke Prevention

Doherty, G. H. 2013. "Homocysteine and Parkinson's disease: A complex relationship." *Journal of Neurologic Disorders* 1: 107.

Garcia-Gracia, C., et al. 2013. "The prevalence of stroke in Parkinson's disease is high: A risk factor assessment." *Neurology* 80: PD 7.033.

Struck, L. K., R. L. Rodnitsky, and J. K. Dobson. 1990. "Stroke and its modification in Parkinson's disease." *Stroke* 21: 1895–99.

Dementia and Cognitive Health

Hendrie, H. C., et al. 2006. "The NIH cognitive and emotional health project: Alzheimer's and dementia." *The Journal of the Alzheimer's Association* 2: 12–32.

Snowdon, D. A., and S. Nun. 2003. "Healthy aging and dementia: Findings from the Nun study." *Annals of Internal Medicine* 139: 450–54.

Williams, J. W., et al. 2010. "Preventing Alzheimer's disease and cognitive decline." In *Evidence Report/Technology Assessment Number 193*. Rockville, MD: Agency for Healthcare Research and Quality, Department of Health and Human.

Balance and Walking

Mancini, F., et al. 2014. "Prevalence and features of peripheral neuropathy in Parkinson's disease patients under different therapeutic regimens." *Parkinsonism and Related Disorders* 20: 27–31.

McGeer, P. L., and E. G. McGeer. 2004. "Inflammation and neurodegeneration in Parkinson's disease." *Parkinsonism and Related Disorders* 10: S3–7.

Rubenstein, L. Z. 2006. "Falls in older people: epidemiology, risk factors, and strategies for prevention." *Age and Ageing* 35 (S2): 37–41.

Shkuratova, N., M. E. Morris, and F. Huxham. 2004. "Effects of age on balance control during walking." *Archives of Physical Medicine and Rehabilitation* 85: 582–88.

Gastrointestinal Health

Cassani, E., et al. 2011. "Use of probiotics for the treatment of constipation in Parkinson's disease patients." *Minerva Gastroenterologica e Dietologica (Journal on Gastroenterology, Nutrition, and Dietetics)* 57: 117–21.

Edwards, L. L., et al. 1991. "Gastrointestinal symptoms in Parkinson's disease." *Movement Disorders* 6: 151–56.

Forsyth, C. B., et al. 2011. "Increased intestinal permeability correlates with sigmoid mucosa alpha-synuclein and endotoxin exposure markers in early Parkinson's disease." *PLoS One* 6(12): e28032. doi:10.1371/journal.pone.0028032

Gabrielli, M., et al. "Prevalence of small intestinal bacterial overgrowth in Parkinson's disease." *Movement Disorders* 26: 889–92.

Pierantozzi, M., et al. 2006. "*Helicobacter pylori* eradication and levodopa absorption in patients with Parkinson's and motor fluctuations." *Neurology* 66: 1824–29.

Skin, Bone, and Dental Health

Bertoni, J. M., et al. 2010. "Increased melanoma risk in Parkinson's disease: A prospective clinicopathological study." *Archives of Neurology* 67: 347–52.

Knekt, P., et al. 2010. "Serum vitamin D and the risk of Parkinson's disease." *JAMA Neurology* 67: 808–11.

Peterson, A. L., et al. 2014. "Memory, mood, and vitamin D in persons with Parkinson's disease." *Journal of Parkinson's Disease* 3: 547–55.

Raglione, L. M., S. Sorbi, and B. Nacmias. 2011. "Osteoporosis and Parkinson's disease." *Clinical Cases in Mineral and Bone Metabolism* 8: 16–18.

CHAPTER 5

Lifestyle Medicine

Lifestyle medicine remains the basic foundation of integrative medicine. It is estimated that more than 70% of illness is caused by or directly influenced by lifestyle, making our everyday decisions some of the most important but often overlooked facets of health. Lifestyle medicine encompasses your habits related to self-care, exercise, diet, and stress management.

WEIGHT MANAGEMENT

The combination of a highly processed, high caloric diet packed with convenience foods and little exercise is leading to a health crisis. The result of this modern-day lifestyle is an increased risk of diabetes, heart disease, high blood pressure, high cholesterol, sleep apnea, cancer, and even brain disease. Obesity is an underlying factor that links these diseases and brain problems such as stroke, dementia, and brain atrophy.

The weight that registers on your scale each morning does not measure the full impact of weight on health. Waist circumference and body mass index (BMI) (defined by weight divided by height) are better predictors of metabolic conditions such as diabetes, heart disease, and even neurodegenerative disease.

Weight gain will affect how you feel with Parkinson's disease (PD), so learning to manage your weight is an important focus of treatment if you are overweight. Symptoms such as fatigue, back and joint pain, sleep apnea, and gastric reflux can increase with added weight. Causes of weight gain in PD include:

- Increased craving for sweets
- Calories from fats and carbohydrates instead of protein[1]
- Reduced exercise
- High intake of high-sugar drinks such as soda and sport drinks
- High intake of coffee and caffeinated drinks for fatigue, often with added sugar and cream
- Increased intake of processed and fast food, if cooking and food preparation are difficult
- Binge eating, which sometimes is a sign of poor impulsivity control associated with dopamine agonists
- Subthalamic nucleus deep brain stimulation (10- to 15-pound average gain)
- Depression

For some, weight loss rather than gain is a serious problem, especially in later stages of the disease, and can be secondary to any of the following:

- Poor appetite
- Loss of smell
- Difficulty chewing
- Increased caloric expenditure from tremor or dyskinesia
- Depression
- Loss of muscle mass
- Nausea caused by dopaminergic medicines

The calories we ingest can potentially influence longevity and brain health. Whether this is also true for PD, however, is far from clear. Animal studies suggest that calorie restriction is associated with reduced effects of aging and increased longevity. These finding have more recently been put to test for PD. Animal studies show that a 30% calorie reduction protected monkeys from dopamine nerve cell damage after injection with a dopamine neurotoxin. This protective effect was associated with increased brain-derived growth factor known to protect nerve cells from cell death. Caloric restriction in rodents also increases levels of glutamate, a neurotransmitter important for movement in PD. Other *theoretical* ways that caloric restriction could help nerve cell function is by lowering oxidative stress from metabolism, reducing protein turnover, and changing levels of neuro-hormones

---

[1] Many people eat less protein since protein reduces levodopa absorption into the bloodstream and brain.

that regulate metabolism. Remember that these are animal studies, and results cannot yet be directly applied to people.

Should Individuals with PD Fast?

At this point the answer is no, since many people with PD suffer from weight loss and/or poor diet. Protein, essential vitamins, and nutrient levels may suffer with a calorie-reduced diet. Lack of energy, fatigue, and loss of muscle mass can impact motor stamina, strength, and motor performance.

Caloric reduction and weight management when needed (under the supervision of an experienced clinician) has many health benefits. Large waist circumference in particular seems to correlate with increased risk of heart disease, diabetes, hypertension, stroke, and even cancer. Of interest is the emerging research showing a link between obesity, marked by abdominal fat (often measured as body mass index or BMI), and brain health. High BMI and waist circumference correlate with lower brain volume in brain regions important to motor, emotional, and cognitive processes. Increase in waist circumference is also associated with changes in regions of the brain that mediate motivational and goal-driven behavior. What's more, the number of dopamine receptors in the striatum (an important structure of the basal ganglia) is reduced when one's waist circumference increases.

People with PD were not included in these studies, so it is not clear if these same results would be noted in this population. What is clear is that weight management is an important goal for overall health if you are overweight with fat accumulation around the waistline. (This finding does not endorse caloric restriction or weight loss in people who are not overweight.) As always, be sure to discuss any changes in diet and weight management with your health care provider. You can find more information about BMI and its calculation in Part V, Personalize Your Care.

TOBACCO AND ALCOHOL USE

Any use of tobacco, whether smoking or chewing, and overuse of alcohol is associated with negative health effects. If you smoke cigarettes or cigars, you are compromising lung function, blood oxygen levels, and the delivery of oxygen to brain cells and increasing oxidative stress and inflammation. Smoking is also a main risk factor for heart disease, stroke, many cancers, and osteoporosis and hip fractures. Smoking will affect how you feel and move with PD as your lung capacity is compromised and stamina and exercise tolerance are decreased.

Epidemiological studies find that smokers have a lower risk of PD even if controlling for age and early death. Of course, this does not mean you should smoke. But this finding has led to additional studies investigating the effect of nicotine on PD.

If you smoke, this is one of the most important lifestyle changes you can make to improve your health. Talk to your doctor about strategies to help you quit. Guided imagery, hypnosis, meditation, exercise, and support and self-help groups are just some of the techniques described in this book that can help you quit smoking. Medical treatments such as nicotine patches/gum, the nicotine blocker varenicline, and the antidepressant bupropion are available to help you deal with cravings.

Unlike smoking, a small amount of alcohol may actually be beneficial to health. Red wine is promoted for its heart and health-promoting effects. Moderate amounts of alcohol reduce heart disease perhaps due to an elevation in HDL (good) cholesterol and reduction in blood clotting. Combined, these changes result in less plaque deposits and blockage in blood vessels, a condition called atherosclerosis. Alcohol can also increases estrogen levels in postmenopausal women, further protecting against heart disease.

The definition of moderate drinking is different for men and women. One four- to six-ounce glass of wine daily may exert health benefits for men compared to one glass three times weekly for women. The drinking guidelines for women are lower in part due to the higher risk of breast cancer associated with more frequent alcohol use in women.

The effect of alcohol on brain health is more complex. Red wine specifically is high in the antioxidant resveratrol, which is under study as a treatment for neurologic conditions such as Alzheimer's disease. Moderate use of alcohol does not affect PD risk but does reduce the risk of developing dementia; however, any amount of alcohol can have negative effects once cognitive decline is present in older persons.

Are the Health Benefits Associated Only with Red Wine, or Are Other Alcoholic Beverages Also Beneficial?

A preliminary study of over 1,000 people with PD showed that drinking one glass of beer daily slightly reduced the risk, but other liquors had the opposite effect. Why beer has a different effect may be related to the fact that beer increases levels of urate, a powerful antioxidant that is currently under study as a neuroprotective agent for PD. Other alcohols also have higher levels of alcohol, which may lead to greater neurotoxic effect. Red wine is particularly high in resveratrol and multiple studies are evaluating its effect on nerve cell health. Overall, these studies are small, and given the known negative effects and addictive potential of alcohol, caution is advised.

Moderation of course is important. Low to moderate use of alcohol is associated with a reduced risk of dementia, but high use can worsen cognitive decline and risk of stroke. Alcohol can increase motor incoordination, imbalance, speech problems, and falls. Alcohol can lower blood pressure, impair sleep, increase confusion and depression, as well as cause withdrawal tremor and other mood problems. Alcohol abuse is often associated with thiamine or vitamin B1 deficiency, a vitamin essential for healthy brain cell function. Alcohol-related liver disease can result in toxic accumulation of ammonia and other chemicals that impact thinking function. Direct toxicity of peripheral nerves and the balance centers of the brain (called the cerebellum) can further impact movement and walking.

Alcohol can also change your daily activity in ways that will influence your well-being. For instance, a glass of wine in the evening may be a nice way to unwind at the end of a busy day. But this may be the only time of day you have to exercise. Or perhaps your habit of nighttime snacking while drinking is not ideal, leading to binges and eating too many unhealthy snacks. These examples serve as an important reminder that moderation and habits change after drinking alcohol. Equally important is how one habit, therapy, or treatment affects other activities. Discuss your alcohol use and potential interactions with medications with your doctor.

EXERCISE

Exercise, once considered a reflection of a person's daily habit, is now an important part of your treatment plan on par with medical therapy. Exercise is important for so many reasons, including:

- General cardiovascular health and stamina
- Disease prevention
- Enhanced motor performance and energy
- Prevention or delay of symptoms associated with disease progression
- Improved PD motor symptoms through neuro-reeducation
- Improved mood, confidence, sleep, and well-being
- Enhanced brain activity through neuroplasticity

There are many different categories of exercise. This list is not exhaustive, but it does represent the more common types of exercise programs studied and/or developed for PD individuals.

- *Aerobic:* exercises that increase heart rate, such as fast-paced walking, jogging, rowing, and cycling
- *Strength:* exercises to strengthen muscles and associated tendons and ligaments for joint stability, such as weight lifting
- *Flexibility:* exercises that increase muscle length and joint flexibility, such as stretching or yoga
- *Agility, balance, and coordination:* exercises that focus on postural alignment, coordination, and graceful flow of sequential movements, such as dance, boxing, and yoga
- *Cognitive-sensory-motor integration:* exercises that use the senses and include cognitive challenges, such as playing computer games, making music, visual targeting, and focusing on body sensations

- *Mind-body:* exercises that combine active engagement of the mind with a focus on breathing, bodily sensations and alignment, imagery, and emotional feelings

What Is the Evidence for Exercise as Medicine for PD?

The physical effects of exercise for people with PD are many, including cardiovascular health, improved lung capacity, increased muscle mass and strength, and bone density. Exercise is also associated with brain changes that include neuroprotection, biochemical alterations, and neuroplasticity.

A meta-analysis, which reviewed the best evidence of multiple PD-associated exercise studies, supports improvement in health-related quality of life, balance, strength, and gait speed. Evidence from this collective analysis did not show that exercise improved depression or reduced falls, however; this could be, in part, due to the lack of carefully designed studies measuring these outcomes. In other words, even exercise—a treatment known to have many positive health-promoting effects—has limited data to support its use in PD (which is the case with other therapies, too). This is not because exercise is ineffective, but because controlled, long-term research studies are often difficult and costly to complete. Despite these limitations, there are a multitude of research findings and observational studies to support the strong ties between PD health and exercise. These findings are discussed in reference to the following outcomes: risk of developing PD, motor symptom control, non-motor symptom control, neuroprotection, and neuroplasticity.

Exercise Reduces the Risk of Developing PD

In a large study analyzing current and prior exercise habits of 48,574 men and 77,254 women, exercise reduced the risk of developing PD. The effect was stronger in men than women and notable for both current exercise regimes and exercise in early adulthood (more than 10 months' strenuous exercise per year). The authors conclude that exercise reduces the risk of developing PD in men or, alternatively, that men at risk tend to exercise less, even years before diagnosis. The later hypothesis could be explained by the possibility that PD-related brain changes are present for decades before the first symptoms are noted and these brain changes can affect activity and behavior. Additional difficulties in drawing more specific conclusions from this study lie in its retrospective nature. Participants were asked to describe their prior exercise activities over many years. This information suffers from accuracy since altered memory and recall bias can influence results.

A more recent study used a prospective approach and followed 43,000 men and women over 12 years as part of the Swedish National March Cohort. None of the participants had PD upon entry into the study and information was obtained from each person about exercise habits, including exercise obtained from daily life chores and occupation and leisure activities. During the time of follow-up,

286 people developed PD. Researchers found that people who spent six hours a day doing physical activity related to household chores or commuting had a 43% reduction in risk compared to those who spent two hours or less daily on these activities. In men, physical activity—defined as 39.1 MET hours[2] per day—was linked to a 45% risk reduction.

Similar to these results, another study showed exercise was linked to a lower risk and another measure, elevated BMI, was linked to a higher risk of PD. Exercise has many effects on the body, including weight loss, so this study illustrates the complex interaction among PD, exercise, and other lifestyle changes.

Moderate-Intensity Exercise

These and other health-related studies show that lifelong exercise is important and the amount needed appears to be moderate in intensity. One way to determine the intensity of a specific task is to use the metabolic equivalent of task (MET) value. The MET value of exercise is less than 3 for light activity, 3 to 6 for moderate activity, and greater than 6 for vigorous activity.

This table describes common daily activities and their MET values per minute; this information will help you understand how much activity is required to reach this MET value.

ACTIVITY	MET/MINUTE
Sleeping	0.9
Walking 2.5 mph, cooking, walking in the house	2–3
Walking one to two blocks or up stairs, raking, gardening, bicycling less than 10 mph	4–5
Golf, singles tennis	6–7
Jumping rope, jogging, swimming, basketball, moderate cycling	8–10
Brisk swimming, running, cross-country skiing, soccer, basketball	10–12
Long-distance running	More than 12

Of course, continued exercise is important after PD. Public health nurses visited and followed 438 patients with PD living in Osaka, Japan, for an average of 4.1 years. Further analysis of this group showed a lower mortality risk for those who exercised compared to those who did not.

Next, we review the effect of exercise on specific motor symptoms, brain physiology, and chemistry.

---

[2] MET hours refers to metabolic equivalent of task, a measure of the energy required to perform physical activity.

Motor Symptom Control

The effect of exercise on PD motor symptoms can be divided into four categories:

- Improved physical performance such as fitness, stamina, and strength
- Improved motor symptoms of bradykinesia, rigidity, speech, and tremor
- Improved motor complications such as "wearing off" effect or dyskinesia
- Improved dopaminergic non-responsive symptoms such as balance, fall risk, and freezing of gait

Improved Physical Performance

Improvement in physical performance means more than improved PD symptoms. Improvement in physical performance relies on improvement in other measures not directly related to the disease, such as muscle strength, stamina, and pulmonary and cardiovascular health. Overall, people with PD tend to exercise less than non-PD individuals and, as a result, they can have lower fitness levels. Fortunately, a lower fitness level is not a given for someone living with PD since regular aerobic exercise can maintain exercise capacity in people with early- to moderate-stage PD as much as those without the disease. Therefore exercise designed to improve strength and endurance is important.

One study measuring the effect of treadmill exercise on walking speed, strength, and fitness revealed interesting results. Three types of exercise performed three times a week over three weeks were tested: high-intensity treadmill, defined as 30 minutes with 70% to 80% heart rate reserve; low-intensity treadmill, defined as 50 minutes at 40% to 50 % heart rate reserve; and a stretching and weight training program. The three exercise routines improved walking speed. As expected, treadmill exercise improved cardiovascular fitness as measured by peak oxygen consumption and strength improved most in the stretching and weight training group. Of interest was the finding that the low-intensity treadmill group (not the high-intensity group) actually had the greatest improvement in gait speed. The reason that the low-intensity workout outperformed the higher-intensity workout in measures of speed is not clear, but explanations include the fact that the low-intensity group walking at a more normal pace could walk longer, which therefore had a greater effect. The other factor could be that fast walking led to a less natural gait or, as the authors noted, "sloppy" or improper walking, and that engaged other brain areas more closely aligned with running than normal walking. It is also possible that the quality of performance, that is, proper body alignment and biomechanics while walking, was important.

It is expected that endurance exercises, such as walking and cycling, can improve the rate of oxygen consumption, a measure of stamina and cardiopulmonary and movement efficiency. Other exercise can also improve exercise tolerance. For instance, yoga practice improved vital capacity in people with PD. Vital capacity is the amount of air expired with a single breath. This important measure not only depends on lung health but also the strength of respiratory muscles and posture, two potential problems in PD. Improved vital capacity could improve ease of breathing with movement and even speech volume, which depends on strong movement of breath while talking. These studies highlight the fact that different exercises will have different performance benefits for people with PD, just as would be expected for the general population and even high-caliber athletes. Often people with PD ask, *"What is the best exercise I can do for my Parkinson's?"* The answer lies not in a single exercise but a multitude of exercises that offer a balance of strength, endurance, and agility.

Improved Motor Symptoms

Exercise can help the PD motor symptoms of rigidity, bradykinesia, and tremor. Many exercise programs have been tested, including physical therapy–guided individualized programs, dance and music programs, yoga, tai chi, treadmill walking, forced exercise, cycling, treadmill walking, weight training, and structured programs such as Feldenkrais Method® and Lee Siverman Voice Treatment (LSVT) Big and Loud®. The degree to which these programs have helped, the specific symptoms that responded best, and the amount of exercise required varies significantly from one study to the next. One of the difficulties in interpreting these studies is the small number of people studied and the limited time of assessment.

Increasing interest surrounds the concept of forced exercise as an ideal exercise for PD. This is based on research observations that high-intensity aerobic exercise designed to increase maximum heart rate improves motor symptoms of PD. Forced exercise, defined as an intensity of 30% greater effort and/or speed than the natural pace for an individual, results in even greater improvement when compared to exercise at the individual's more natural preferred rate. Initial studies should be interpreted with caution, since they are small in number of participants, tend to include early disease, and researchers were not blinded to the treatment group and therefore subject to bias. A blinded study is one in which the investigators performing the study and the subjects are blinded or unaware if treatment is real or placebo. Forced exercise can be achieved by increasing speed on the treadmill or exercise bike. A personal trainer is especially helpful to push intensity beyond a natural speed. This exercise paradigm should be supervised by a clinical specialist to ensure safety especially in people with heart or lung disease, diabetes, or low blood pressure.

Intensity has been shown to improve neuroplasticity and enhance motor outcomes. It should be noted that although high-intensity exercise is beneficial, there are many other aspects of exercise tied to neuroplasticity that could have equal or complementary benefits. The treadmill study described previously, showing "normal"-paced treadmill walkers outperforming fast-paced treadmill walkers, reinforces the argument that quality may be better than quantity.

Improved Motor Complications

Mid- to late-stage PD is associated with motor fluctuations and dyskinesia. The most common form of motor fluctuation is end-of-dose "wearing off" effect. This describes the return of motor symptoms when medicine benefits wear off and, in turn, improvement of motor symptoms after medication dosage is taken. Motor fluctuation, or *on-off* periods, can also be associated with dyskinesia, most commonly as a medication peak dose effect. Dyskinesia is experienced as uncontrollable involuntary movement such as twisting, writing, swaying, and bobbing.

It is helpful to time your exercise to avoid the medicine off-state, if possible. Increased muscle rigidity, dystonia, reduced joint range of motion, and motor agility can all impact one's ability to exercise and impair the quality of performance. Other factors such as motor fatigue, motivation, mood, and attention can fluctuate with on-off periods and impact one's exercise abilities.

Dyskinesia can sometimes increase with exercise and impair the ability to exercise. Factors other than medicine timing that can worsen dyskinesia include stress and movement challenge. In other words, exercise that is more difficult to perform or requires multitasking or learning could potentially worsen dyskinesia. Exercises that promote relaxation, such as music therapy and yoga, can potentially help dyskinesia through this indirect effect.

People with PD may ask, *"Can exercise actually improve dyskinesia?"* The answer to this question will vary from individual to individual. One way that exercise can potentially help dyskinesia is to directly target the factors known to increase this problem. Exercise designed to reduce fatigue, anxiety, or fear and enhance motor confidence and performance could improve dyskinesia. Whether there is a more direct connection between exercise and the pathologic brain changes associated with dyskinesia is unclear. At least one study directly examined the effect of rehabilitation therapy on dyskinesia and proved that an intensive inpatient physical and occupational therapy program could improve dyskinesia, but this effect may be due to reduced medication dosage over the course of the study.

Improved Dopaminergic Nonresponsive Symptoms

Some PD motor symptoms may not improve with dopaminergic medicine. These symptoms of more advanced disease include balance, postural changes, speech, and swallowing problems. Flexed posture affects breathing, walking speed, balance, and shoulder range of motion. Abnormal posture can worsen pain from spine disease or arthritis and even affect confidence and social interactions. The effect of exercise on posture is rarely discussed, but exercise can make a difference. Spine or truncal flexibility did improve after a physical therapy–guided, 10-week flexibility and training program.

Exercise focused on the problem you are having can help. For instance, walking and leg strengthening exercises will improve walking speed. Targeted balance exercises will improve balance. Exercise programs associated with notable improvement in balance include tai chi and tango dancing. In research studies, changes in walking and balance are analyzed by timed tasks, rating scales, and questionnaires. Although these are important measures, they do not measure the specific problem of walking, balance, or fall risk that you face in your home's natural environment. Of utmost importance to individuals with PD is the distance they can comfortably walk (endurance), walking-associated falls, and fear of falling or near falls. One particular problem, freezing of gait (FoG) or difficulties initiating first steps when walking, is a troublesome symptom that can lead to falls.

The severity of FoG is caused by many factors, including disease response to medications (FoG most often does not improve with levodopa and is present in the motor on- or off-state, but in milder cases may be experienced only in the medicine off-state), crowded and cluttered environments, anxiety, and cognitive or motor challenges. The majority of work on FoG has focused on cueing strategies with notable benefit. Cueing is the use of sensory or cognitive strategies to improve motor initiation. Examples include using visual targets, such as lines on the floor or visual imagery, tapping, or music.

The effect of exercise on falls and FoG, however, is less predictable. A recent study highlights this finding. A three times weekly 40- to 60-minute exercise program, undertaken for six months, improved balance, mobility, quality of life, fear of falls, and mood yet did not improve rate of falls. This discrepancy is in part due to the many factors that contribute to falls that would be difficult to control for in a research study including impulsivity, fatigue and weakness, stamina, change in activity level with improved well-being, anxiety, fear, environment, and even use of proper footwear. For instance, improved measures of walking and balance must be accompanied by improvement in strength, confidence, stamina, attention, and judgment to have the greatest impact on fall risk. FoG, a main contributor of falls, depends on proper medicine dosing and is greatly influenced by the environment. Finally, increased falls could be the result of improved mobility, which brings improved confidence and increased physical activity, risk taking, and exploration of new physical tasks or challenges.

Non-Motor Symptoms

The following list includes many of the non-motor symptoms that could potentially improve with exercise.

- General
  - Fatigue and energy
  - General confidence
  - Improved global measures of quality of life
  - Socialization
  - Pain

- Cognitive
  - Improved executive dysfunction and attention skills

- Behavior
  - Mood and depression
  - Anxiety
  - Confidence
  - Sleep

- Autonomic control
  - Constipation
  - Orthostatic hypotension (dizziness with standing)

Specific exercises that target these symptoms include high-intensity aerobic exercise to improve cognitive abilities and mood disorders. Sensorimotor and mind-body exercises are particularly helpful for cognitive and behavioral symptoms. Orthostatic hypotension can worsen with intense exercise and is best treated with a gradual exercise program, beginning with exercise in the lying or seated position and focusing on specific leg movements to increase venous blood flow in the legs. Be sure to work with a specialist if you have orthostatic hypotension. Exercise that is performed incorrectly, fast movement, and movement that increases abdominal pressure can worsen blood pressure fluctuations.

A note of caution: Exercise can lead to dehydration due to fluid loss from increased breathing and sweating. Be sure to drink plenty of fluids when exercising to avoid dizziness, low blood pressure, and problems with constipation that can accompany PD.

Neuroprotection

Neuroprotection is a form of neuroplasticity of particular importance to PD. Neuroprotection, simply described, is the protection of vulnerable nerve cells at risk for damage, degeneration, or decline with disease. Neuroprotection in PD is defined as the protection of dopamine nerve cells in the basal ganglia from future loss or cell death.

Animal models of PD are ideally suited to measure the neuroprotective effects of exercise. In these studies, neurotoxins are delivered to animals. One particular neurotoxin, 6-OHDA, causes dopamine nerve cell death in rodents. This nerve cell loss is associated with motor problems such as slowness, impaired coordination, and decreased walking speed. Both dopamine nerve cell loss and the movement changes associated with loss of dopamine activity are reduced by exercise. This protective effect was seen when exercise was initiated at the timing of neurotoxin exposure and when it preceded the exposure.

Studying neuroprotection in people is much more difficult. What is known is that exercise reduces the risk of PD, improves motor symptoms, enhances cognitive performance and other non-motor symptoms, and appears to modify symptom progression. Whether this is due to the influence of exercise on general health and cerebrovascular health, associated positive lifestyle change, increased strength and enhanced motor performance, a direct dopamine neuroprotective effect, increased efficacy of neurochemical release, or more generalized positive neuroplasticity is unknown. What is clear is that exercise truly influences current and future symptoms of PD. A graduated and balanced exercise program that increases the intensity or challenge over time should be coupled with optimal medical treatment to achieve the best results.

Neuroplasticity

We have already reviewed the importance of neuroplasticity or the brain's ability to change in response to activity and experience. Exercise-induced neuroplasticity and/or associated neuroprotection in PD is an active area of research and personal interest. Similar to other activities, the type and quality of exercise appears to influence the type and quality of neuroplasticity. The following exercise qualities appear to be important:

- *Intensity.* These exercises could include aerobic exercise performed with enhanced effort.
- *Specificity.* These exercises are specific to the intended goal. Examples are walking and balance activities to improve walking performance.
- *Difficulty.* These exercises are more difficult tasks that require skill acquisition and learning.
- *Complexity.* These exercises could include movements that require complex motor choreography or rely on sensory and cognitive integration, such as yoga or dance.
- *Value and meaning.* These exercises are associated with positive and meaningful experiences and might include activities influenced by the effect of music, social integration, personal passion, and enjoyment.

In effect, positive and generalized neuroplasticity can be achieved through a well-rounded and balanced approach with exercises performed in each of the aforementioned categories. Tango dancing, a form of exercise proven to improve balance in people with PD, may have this effect simply because this form of dance requires precise change in speed, direction, and center of gravity. Tango does indeed have a certain degree of intensity, difficulty, and motor complexity. Of broader importance is the dancer's entire experience of tango. The following qualities may further expand tango's neuroplastic potential. Tango dancing is:

- Socially engaging and interactive
- Intimate, involving touch and an emotional connection with your partner
- Musical and upbeat
- Emotionally uplifting
- Sensorimotor integration through touch and music
- Cognitively challenging

Neurochemistry

The effect of exercise on neurochemistry or brain neurotransmitter levels is yet one more way that exercise can influence neuroplasticity and PD motor symptoms. High-intensity treadmill and cycling are associated with dopaminergic brain changes that mimic those seen after medication. Treadmill or high-intensity exercise also increases the efficiency by which nerve cells use dopamine. It is important to note that exercise is not intended to replace medication. More important, dopaminergic medicine can improve the ability to perform and experience "normal" movement, which is important for neuroplasticity. Exercise can also help produce a more natural chemical balance by influencing how brain cells use dopamine.

Personalized Exercise Prescription

The type of exercise for PD health depends on the goals. A balanced approach will include aerobic exercise, posture and balance work, resistance (strength) training, flexibility, agility, motor learning, and personal meaning. Some exercise programs target just one of these areas while others target many of these exercise goals. Researchers have found the following exercises or programs to be helpful for PD:

- *Walking and balance:* dance, tango, treadmill, aerobics, tai chi
- *Tremor:* treadmill, cycling, mindfulness movement
- *Cognition:* aerobic exercise, sensorimotor integration
- *Mood:* aerobic exercise, yoga, tai chi

Choose exercises or activities you enjoy and that are challenging and perhaps new to you, requiring you to learn new movements. Consider beginning with a physical therapist to reduce risk of injury and avoid becoming overwhelmed by the many exercise programs available. Choosing the best exercise is simple: it's the exercise that you will continue to do. Find ways to keep yourself motivated. Setting and recording goals, using DVDs, exercising with others in a class, using the buddy system, personal coaches and trainers, computer programs, and smartphone apps are just some of the techniques or strategies that can keep you on track.

An exercise inventory is included in Part V, Personalize Your Care, to help you set your personal exercise routine.

INTERVIEW WITH THE EXPERT: EXERCISE, PHYSICAL THERAPISTS, AND PERSONAL TRAINERS

At what stage should a person with Parkinson's seek therapies?

People with PD should establish their health care team as soon as possible after diagnosis. The health care team should involve rehabilitation professionals who may include physical, occupational, and speech-language pathologists. Consulting with the rehabilitation

(continued)

INTERVIEW WITH THE EXPERT (*continued*)

team early is important because a focus on prevention is often the best medicine. If challenges do arise, seeking rehabilitation treatment early can help prevent further decline. Getting educated on rehabilitation options and engaging in treatment promptly can optimize health benefits and overall wellness while reducing disability over time.

How would therapy differ in early disease vs. later disease?

Early in the disease process, therapy will focus on prevention and wellness. Since the challenges people with PD face over the course of the disease are known, therapy can target these areas (i.e., mobility, speech) early with the goal of preventing or slowing decline. Once challenges arise, therapy focuses on **remediation**, or improving the underlying problems. Over time, therapy may focus on **compensation**, or adapting to the problem by identifying alternate solutions to improve function. Therapy is beneficial at all stages of the disease; however, early intervention is recommended to optimize outcome.

Are there specific types of physical therapy for Parkinson's?

Research studies reveal that physical therapy in the form of exercise can improve walking, balance, fitness, strength, and flexibility in persons with PD. There is no one type of exercise that has been shown to be more beneficial than another. An optimal exercise program incorporates elements of aerobic conditioning, strength training, balance, and flexibility exercises. There are various options available to incorporate these elements into an exercise program. For example, brisk walking or cycling will provide benefits of aerobic conditioning. Strength training can be carried out using weight machines, dumbbells, or resistance bands. Tai chi or dance classes may improve balance. LSVT Big and Loud® training may improve the amplitude or size of movements. The good news is that people with PD have a variety of options to choose from. Incorporating the important elements of exercise on different days of the week may optimize the benefit. For example, aerobic conditioning may be a focus of an exercise program on a few days of the week, whereas balance and strengthening exercises may be the focus on different days.

(continued)

INTERVIEW WITH THE EXPERT (*continued*)

This way, all the important elements of exercise can be included. Long-term engagement in regular exercise is the key to success. Choosing exercise options that are most enjoyable is the best way to stick to a program over time.

How is a physical therapist different from a personal trainer?

People with PD may benefit from working with physical therapists and personal trainers, but it is important to understand how their roles differ. Physical therapists are highly educated, licensed *health care* professionals who provide rehabilitation to patients with a variety of health conditions to help improve or restore mobility, increase function, and reduce disability. Physical therapists provide health care services for people in a variety of settings, including hospitals, private practices, outpatient clinics, home health agencies, schools, sports and fitness facilities, work settings, and nursing homes. Physical therapy services are typically reimbursed in part or in full by a variety of health insurance companies including Medicare. Personal trainers, on the other hand, are fitness professionals who work with the general, healthy population to develop an exercise program to improve fitness. They help clients set fitness-related goals and provide motivation, feedback, and accountability. They typically work in health and fitness centers and are most often paid privately as an out-of-pocket expense.

Is there benefit in having a physical therapist and personal trainer working together?

There is a benefit when physical therapists and personal trainers work together to help meet the needs of persons with PD. A physical therapist is knowledgeable about health conditions, such as PD, and can conduct an initial examination of functional ability (e.g., walking, moving in bed, rising from sitting to standing) to determine the nature of any limitations (i.e., strength, aerobic conditioning, balance and flexibility) in order to optimize mobility and participation in desired activities (i.e., work, travel, socialization, recreational activities). The physical therapist will develop an individualized exercise program tailored to address any challenges or limitations identified during the examination. To optimize outcome, the exercise

(*continued*)

INTERVIEW WITH THE EXPERT (*continued*)

program must be implemented on a regular basis over the course of a lifetime! This is where working with a personal trainer can be beneficial. Physical therapists and personal trainers can partner to help people with PD carry out their exercise programs routinely. A personal trainer might attend a physical therapy session with a person with PD or talk to a physical therapist by phone to discuss the plan for exercise. The personal trainer can learn the optimal exercises specifically tailored to individuals with PD in addition to those exercises to avoid, reducing risk of injury. Individuals can then set up a schedule to work with a personal trainer to establish an exercise routine. Regular follow-up appointments with a physical therapist (approximately every six months) are recommended to reassess functional mobility and determine if modifications to the exercise program are needed. This partnership provides a wellness-oriented approach to help reduce disability, achieve long-term health benefits, and improve quality of life.

Terry Ellis, PT, PhD, NCS
Assistant Professor
Director, Center for Neurorehabilitation
Boston University

NUTRITION

One of the most common questions I am asked is, *"What diet should I follow?"* Whether it is the foods we choose, how it is grown, or how it is prepared, what we eat affects health.

Eating well does not mean following the latest diet craze claiming fast results to weight loss, energy, or cure of disease. Eating well means making the right food choices to ensure you get the appropriate vitamins and nutrients and to reduce your risk of cardiovascular disease, hypertension, diabetes, obesity, intestinal problems, stroke, and cancer.

There is no specific diet for PD, but there are sound guidelines that can serve you well. We will review the basic science of nutrition before diving into a review of more popular diets touted for their health effects.

Food chemistry can be divided into two categories: macronutrients and micronutrients. Macronutrients are the major food categories of carbohydrates, fats, proteins, and fiber. Micronutrients are vitamins and substances found in food and needed in smaller amounts to promote cell health and catalyze biochemical reactions.

Carbohydrates

Most of us are familiar with carbohydrates as a quick energy source due to their efficient use by our bodies. Carbohydrates can be divided into simple sugars, complex carbohydrates, and starches based on their chemical structure. These differences also mean that they are processed differently by the body, so all carbohydrates should not be treated the same.

Simple Sugars. Simple sugars are made up of one or two sugar units. Glucose is the most important sugar unit used to fuel cells and the primary energy source for brain cells. Your body will produce glucose from protein when glucose levels are low and not replenished through food. Examples of simple sugars are:

- One sugar unit: glucose, fructose (fruits), and galactose, which are absorbed quickly since they do not require digestion
- Two sugar units
  - Lactose (present in milk) = glucose and galactose
  - Sucrose (table sugar) = glucose and fructose
  - Maltose = glucose and glucose

Complex Carbohydrates. Complex carbohydrates consist of long chains of sugar molecules linked together like beads on a necklace. Complex carbohydrates can be divided into forms that are digestible and those that are not, as follows:

- *Starch:* A long chain of carbohydrate that is digestible by the body. Starches must be metabolized before being absorbed so they do not cause as fast a rise in glucose as simple sugars.
- *Fiber:* A form of carbohydrate that is resistant to metabolic breakdown in the intestinal tract.

There is a tremendous amount of information warning of the perils of sugar and carbohydrates and often conflicting guidance about which carbohydrates or how much to eat. Like everything else, the quality of carbohydrate is important. This is not simply a matter of whether the carbohydrate is a simple or complex sugar. One way to measure a food's carbohydrate quality is the glycemic index or glycemic load. These are measures of a food's tendency to increase blood glucose levels after ingestion, as follows:

- *Glycemic Index[3]:* The glycemic index is a ranking of carbohydrates based on how quickly sugar is absorbed into the bloodstream. It is measured on a scale of 0 to 100, with 100 set as the index for glucose. Foods with lower numbers are better than foods with a higher index.
- *Glycemic Load (GL):* GL is the glycemic index of the food multiplied by the amount of carbohydrate in food. A GL greater than 20 is considered high. Learn more about the GL of common foods in Part V, Personalize Your Care.

---

[3] More information on the glycemic index of foods is available at www.glycemicindex.com

Foods with a higher GL lead to a more rapid increase in blood sugar after they are eaten. These measures are a better measure of a food's impact on blood sugar levels than whether a food is designated a simple or complex carbohydrate, since there are other factors that influence a food's GL. These factors include how it is processed, prepared, the serving size, and the foods it is eaten with. Puffed, blended, crushed, or refined foods have a higher surface-to-volume ratio, allowing faster digestion and absorption than whole foods. Foods cooked until soft have a higher load than if cooked al dente. Finally, sweets will have a higher GL when eaten alone compared to when paired with other foods high in fat, fiber, or protein. The following examples illustrate these points:

- Puffed white rice has a higher index than white rice. But since less puffed rice is eaten compared to white rice, the GL is lower.
- Watermelon has a high glycemic index of 72 but a low GL of 3.6, since there is a lot of water and fiber in one slice or serving.
- White potatoes have higher GLs than sweet potatoes because of the higher fiber in sweet potatoes.
- Oranges have a lower GL than orange juice because juice from one orange has less pulp and fiber than an orange. Add to this the fact that many people drink more juice than that squeezed from one orange.
- Gluten-free bread may have a greater GL than a non-gluten product, since it often has less fiber and protein.
- The GL of a sweet desert is higher when eaten alone as a snack than when eaten after a meal or snack with protein or fiber.

CLINICAL PEARL: MORE ABOUT GL

GL is the measure of the amount that a given food or meal will increase blood glucose levels. One unit is equivalent to the effect of eating one gram of glucose. The GL ranges from 0 to 100. A number less than 20 is low and greater than 20 is high.

$$\text{Glycemic Load} = \text{Glycemic Index} \times \text{Amount of carbohydrate in a serving}$$

The effect of sugar on the body is complex. These tips will help you reduce your diet's GL.

- Chose whole fruits and vegetables over blended, juiced, or processed foods.

(continued)

CLINICAL PEARL (*continued*)

- Choose complex carbohydrates and whole grains such as oats, rye, barely, brown rice, wheat berries, beans, and quinoa over refined grains.
- Increase consumption of foods high in fiber since high fiber from whole grains, fruits, and vegetables will reduce GL.
- Eat small portions of sweets, and eat them as part of a balanced meal rather than alone as a snack.
- Avoid highly processed foods and high fructose sweetener and choose instead foods that are "close to the earth"—that is, foods that are in their natural state with little to no processing.
- Combine foods high in water, fiber, and protein to reduce the GL.
- Add lemon juice, vinegar, and fermented foods to your meal to reduce GL.
- Add cinnamon to desserts since it has been shown to slow absorption of glucose.
- Eat fresh foods in their natural state for snacks instead of processed, blended, or pulverized foods.

Of course, sugary processed foods such as cookies, pies, cakes, soda, sweetened drinks, and sugary syrups should be avoided or eaten in small portions. The following list highlights carbohydrates that have a lower GL than their counterparts, as well as other "PD friendly" foods that are also low on the GL index:

Carbohydrates

- Pumpernickel, rye, sourdough, and grainy, nutty whole wheat in place of white bread
- Quinoa, millet, bulgur, bran, farro, barley, couscous, and brown rice instead of white rice
- Al dente in place of overcooked pasta
- Whole wheat pasta over white pasta
- Sweet potatoes in place of white potatoes

Fiber

- Oatmeal, a good source of soluble fiber

(*continued*)

CLINICAL PEARL (continued)

Healthy Fats

- Olives, high in antioxidants and healthy fats
- Avocado, high in antioxidants and healthy fats
- Nuts, high in antioxidants, fiber, and healthy fats

Protein

- Nuts, a non-animal source of protein and antioxidants
- Black and kidney beans, a non-animal source of protein and high in antioxidants

Antioxidants

- *Fruits.* Some fruits are high in glucose and low in fiber or fluid. This combination increases GL. Examples include papaya, melons, mango, and pineapple. Choose low GL fruits such as blueberries, raspberries, grapefruit, grapes, and citrus.
- *Vegetables.* Most vegetables are lower in GL. Vegetables with higher GL are still healthy but should be eaten in moderation. Examples include carrots, potatoes, peas, and winter squash. Otherwise choose low GL vegetables such as peppers, onions, cucumbers, green leafy vegetables, and broccoli.

Fats

Fats are a necessary part of our diet. Naturally occurring fats are divided into three types:

- Saturated fats
- Monounsaturated fats
- Polyunsaturated fats

Saturated Fats. These fats are solid at room temperature and are found primarily in red meat, tropical oils such as coconut, avocado, and dairy products. A diet high in saturated fats (notably from animal sources) can increase cholesterol levels.

Monounsaturated Fats. These fats are liquid at room temperature but get cloudy when refrigerated. Examples of monounsaturated fats include olives and olive oil, canola oil, nuts and nut oils, and avocado. These oils are a better substitute for saturated fats, can reduce cholesterol levels, and improve insulin activity.

Polyunsaturated Fats. These fats are liquid both at room temperature and when refrigerated. Polyunsaturated fats can be divided into two types: omega-6 and omega-3. Omega-6 fats include sunflower oil, safflower oil, corn oil, most seeds, and oil from grains. Omega-3 fats are found in walnuts, flaxseed, pumpkin seeds, purslane, and cold water fish such as salmon, tuna, and sardines. Omega-3 fats are found in highest concentration in the brain and are important to brain cell function.

Omega-6 fats will increase inflammation in the body when eaten in excess of omega-3 fatty acids. The American diet is high in omega-6 relative to omega-3 fat largely from processed foods—sometimes up to five times more than the recommended ratio of 2:1 or 4:1 omega-6 to omega-3. Increasing intake of omega-3 relative to omega-6 foods can reduce cellular inflammation and your risk of heart disease, certain cancers, depression, stroke, dementia, and asthma.

There are no data, to date, showing that omega-3 supplements (fish oil) reduce PD risk or symptoms. However, diets and cell levels high in omega-3 may have more generalized positive brain effects. Diets high in omega-3 are associated with larger brain volume in the hippocampus, an important part of the brain involved in learning. Other ways that omega-3s can help brain health is through reduced inflammation and lipid peroxidation (a form of oxidative stress).

Recommendations: Avoid trans and hydrogenated fats (read your food labels) often found in processed and fast foods. Reduce your saturated fats by limiting the amount of red meat you eat to twice or less weekly. Choose low-fat milk and dairy products. Use olive oil for cooking and salad dressings instead of corn oil and other oils high in omega-6. Aim for two servings of cold water fish weekly. Add whole nuts, avocados, and olives to your diet.

CLINICAL PEARL: HIGH FRUCTOSE SWEETENER AND HYDROGENATED FATS

High fructose sweetener and hydrogenated fats are examples of chemically modified ingredients added to foods to increase their shelf life, consistency, and sweetness.

Hydrogenated Oils and Trans-Fat. These fats are made by adding hydrogen to oils to saturate chemical bonds. The resultant fats are solid at room temperature. These fats do not spoil as fast and add a creamy consistency to foods. Trans-fats increase blood levels of bad cholesterol (LDL) and decrease good cholesterol (HDL), increasing

(*continued*)

CLINICAL PEARL (*continued*)

risk of heart disease and stroke. Examples of common foods that contain these types of fats are:

- Shortening and margarine
- Nondairy creamers and whipped toppings
- Fried foods, cookies, pastry
- Peanut butter and frostings
- Snack chips, crackers, microwave popcorn

High Fructose Corn Syrup (HFCS). HFCS is produced chemically from corn, resulting in a glucose-to-fructose ratio of 45:55 (unlike table sugar, which is 50:50). The fructose is much sweeter than glucose, which is appealing to many palates. However, absorption of fructose through the gastrointestinal (GI) tract is slower and requires more chemical energy. Increased exposure of GI cells to fructose in turn may change the integrity of cells lining the GI tract and potentially lead to problems with a leaky gut. Plus, foods with HFCS are of poor quality with little nutritional benefits.

The following suggestions can help you avoid these artificial products when possible:

- Read food labels.
- Eat whole foods such as fruit instead of processed desserts and drinks.
- Use olive oil, avocado oil, and even butter in place of margarine, shortening, or mayonnaise.
- Look for natural peanut butter and use fruit spread instead of jellies and jams.
- Avoid sweetened sodas and syrups.

Proteins

Proteins are needed for wound healing and cell and muscle growth. Amino acids, the building blocks of protein, are used in the formation of antioxidants such as glutathione, synthesis of neurotransmitters, and synthesis of glucose. A diet too high in protein can lead to bone loss and may be harmful to persons with kidney disease. A diet too low in protein can produce anemia and affect immune health and muscle stores.

Essential amino acids are amino acids that cannot be synthesized by the body and can only be obtained from foods. Complete proteins are foods that include all essential amino acids. Meat, dairy, and eggs are essential amino acids while many plant-based proteins are not. Quinoa and soy are plants that are complete proteins. Combination foods such as rice and beans are a complete source of protein when eaten together. The American guidelines for protein are 0.8 gm/kg body weight (0.36 gm/pound). You may need more protein if you are vegetarian, suffering from infection, or recovering from an injury.

Protein can delay the absorption of levodopa (found in Sinemet®, Rytary®, or Stalevo®) into the bloodstream and across the blood-brain barrier into the brain. This is not the case for medicines that do not include levodopa. This is less of a problem with mild PD but can be more of an issue in advancing disease in which fluctuations or dyskinesia are present. Interference is greater with meat proteins than plant proteins. This is due to the fact that meat protein is more slowly absorbed than plant proteins.

Recommendations: Do not avoid protein for fear that it will interfere with your medicines since protein is a necessary nutrient for health. Try to take levodopa one hour before or after meals to improve the absorption of this medicine. If you are taking frequent doses of levodopa and this recommendation is too difficult, then you can try to eat the majority (70%) of your protein in the evening or alternately eat small amounts of protein frequently throughout the day instead of just two to three times daily. Increase the amount of protein you get each week from fish and plant-based sources by reducing your intake of red meat to once weekly and increasing fish to twice weekly. Plant protein is ideal since plants are usually high in fiber, complex carbohydrates, antioxidants, and low in saturated fats. Examples of plant-based proteins are:

- Nuts
- Beans
- Soy, tempeh, and tofu
- Quinoa
- Green leafy vegetables, such as spinach and broccoli
- Chia and hemp seeds
- Seitan, which is made from seasoned gluten as a meat substitute
- Lentils
- Chickpeas and hummus
- Greek yogurt

Fiber

Unlike starch, fiber is not digested by the body. There are two types of fiber: soluble and insoluble. Soluble fiber dissolves in water and can slow gastric emptying and cause you to feel full. Examples include many fruits, flax, oatmeal, and psyllium (Metamucil®). Insoluble fiber found in vegetables, whole grains, raisins, and prunes does not absorb water and passes through the GI tract to aid motility and reduce constipation.

Fiber is an important treatment for constipation, so often a problem for people with PD. The recommended daily intake of fiber is 20 to 30 grams daily.

Recommendations: A diet of fresh fruits, vegetables, and whole grains with infrequent consumption of sugary processed foods, desserts, and drinks offers the healthiest carbohydrates and highest fiber.

PD Food Pyramid

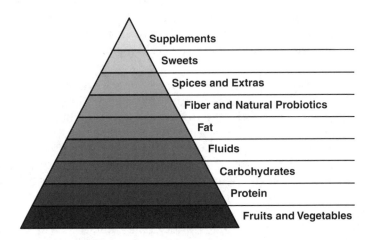

Supplements
Sweets
Spices and Extras
Fiber and Natural Probiotics
Fat
Fluids
Carbohydrates
Protein
Fruits and Vegetables

Fruits and Vegetables

Aim for 8 to 10 servings a day that are:

- High in antioxidants to maintain a healthy body and brain cells. No single antioxidant is best. A variety of antioxidants in your diet will lead to better protection against oxidative stress. Eat fruits and vegetables in a variety of colors to ensure a variety of antioxidants.
- High in fiber for colon health and to reduce constipation.
- Natural sources of high-quality carbohydrates for energy.

Protein

Select vegetable protein as your major source, followed in frequency by fish, dairy (or a dairy substitute such as soy), then meat.

Vegetable proteins (beans, nuts, seeds, and quinoa) have these benefits:

- Low in saturated fat and better for heart and brain health.
- High in fiber, resulting in better colon health and reduced constipation.
- High in antioxidants.
- Cause less interference with levodopa absorption than animal protein.

Fish and seafood:

- Lower in saturated fat than other forms of protein.
- High in omega-3 "good fats," which are needed for a healthy heart and brain and are shown to improve many conditions. Cold water fish is especially healthy to eat.

Dairy or dairy substitute (soy):

- Both are sources of calcium, important for strong bones.
- Choose low-fat milk without hormones or additives to reduce intake of saturated fat.
- Consider the use of soy or other vegetable-based milk products in place of dairy because some studies suggest dairy products increase the risk of PD.

Carbohydrates

Whole grains are better than premade processed foods. Increase carbohydrates in the form of starchy vegetables, beans, and whole grains.

- Improved glucose control means better health and perhaps better aging!
- These foods adds fiber, other nutrients, and antioxidants.

Limit processed sugars high in fat and refined sugar since they:

- Have limited balanced nutritional value, meaning you get less protein, fiber, vitamins, minerals, and antioxidants yet get all the calories.
- Lead to fluctuations in energy levels and fatigue.

Fluids

- Water is needed to prevent dehydration, low blood pressure, and dizziness, and it helps with constipation.
- Fruit and vegetable juices are good choices, but talk to your doctor about sugar and salt levels in these beverages.
- Coffee and green and white tea are high in antioxidants, but excessive caffeine can increase tremor and insomnia. Choose decaffeinated brands.

Fat

A small amount of the right kinds of fats are good.

- Choose foods rich in omega-3 fatty acids, such as salmon, sardines, flaxseed, and walnuts.
- Olive oil can be used instead of other cooking or salad oils.
- Coconut oil is high in medium-chain fatty acids and easy to cook with.

Fiber and Natural Probiotics

These foods are important for colon health and constipation.

- Fiber comes from many sources, but many of us have trouble getting enough. Fiber-rich foods include fruits, vegetables, nuts, whole grains, and oats.
- Natural probiotics can reduce GI inflammation and reduce symptoms of constipation. Examples include pickled and fermented foods such as sauerkraut, kombucha, kefir, and yogurt. Talk to your doctor before adding these foods if you have immune system problems.

Spices and Extras

- Green tea.
- Spices with antioxidants and anti-inflammatory properties include turmeric, garlic, and cinnamon.
- Alcohol. Although one glass of red wine is sometimes recommended due to the health benefits of the powerful antioxidant resveratrol, it can interact with PD medicine and worsen balance, lightheadedness, and confusion.

Sweets

Many people with PD have a sweet tooth. If you do not have diabetes, it is okay to enjoy sweets but sparingly. If you take in too many calories with sweets you do not get the vitamins, minerals, and nutrients you need for health.

- Fruit desserts and fruit smoothies made with real fruit will help you get your extra fruit servings.
- The flavinoids in dark chocolate (more than 70% cocoa) is a strong antioxidant and good for mood, too!

Supplements

Talk to your doctor about the following supplements:

- Multivitamin
- Fiber supplement
- Fish oil
- Coenzyme Q10
- Calcium
- Vitamin D
- B12

Food and Parkinson's

There is no food or diet proven to slow the progression of PD. There are, however, foods that are associated with an increased and reduced risk of developing

PD. The following table lists foods or diets found to influence PD risk and possible reasons why.

INCREASED RISK	DECREASED RISK	PROPOSED REASON(S)
Milk (not cheese or yogurt)		Low urate levels; pesticide or other chemical contaminates may contribute to cell damage
Diet high in meat		Excess iron in heme (red meat) may contribute to cell damage
	Prudent diet* Mediterranean diet	High in antioxidants, low in inflammatory fats and processed sugars
	Beta carotene (carrots)	Antioxidant
	Peppers	High nicotine levels may protect nerve cells
	Berries	Antioxidant (anthocyanins)
	Coffee	Antioxidant, adenosine blockade
	Green tea	Antioxidant

*A diet high in fruit, vegetable, and fish intake.

Diets

Mediterranean diet. Adherence to the Mediterranean diet is associated with a lower risk of PD (14% to 48%) and later age of disease onset. Similar studies suggest a lower risk between a similar prudent diet compared with the Western diet. This finding is further strengthened by consistent findings that the Mediterranean diet is proven to reduce the risk of so many other diseases such as stroke, depression, dementia, hypertension, heart disease, diabetes, and cancer, proving its global impact on health and disease.

Recommendations are to eat a diet that is:

- High in fruits and vegetables, with 8 to 10 servings daily
- High in fish, two to three times per week
- Low in red meat, one to two times week
- High in plant protein
- High in whole grains
- Low in processed refined sugar

In addition, the Mediterranean diet uses olive oil as a primary oil and allows moderate amounts of red wine.

There are other diets popular with people with PD, but there is no evidence to support the benefits of these diets over the prudent diet recommendations. Of course, adherence to any diet is usually associated with improved well-being perhaps due to greater attention to food selection and preparation, intentional planning of meals, and wiser choices, such as fewer processed and fast foods. Also healthy habits in one area such as diet often influence other habits or other healthy activities such as exercise.

Paleolithic diet. This diet focuses on foods available to our hunter and gatherer ancestors over 10,000 years ago, such as meat, eggs, fruits, berries, and certain vegetables, especially root vegetables. Foods to avoid with this diet are potatoes, sugar, dairy, and grains. There is an assumption that our diets do not match our genetic and environmental biology, which is certain to be the case. However, the assumption that the best match lies in the much-distant Paleolithic era is a major yet unproven assumption. It is also questionable as to whether the agriculturally raised meat, eggs, and produce of today are similar to that in the past. The elimination of potential neurotoxins present in foods and lower ingestion of foods with high GL is the rationale behind this low carbohydrate diet. Certainly this is also the objective of the prudent diet. There is no evidence that this high fat, moderate protein, low carbohydrate Paleolithic diet alters PD risk or that it is superior to the prudent diet.

Gluten-free diet. Celiac disease is an autoimmune disorder found in 1% of the population. Ingestion of gluten, a protein found in wheat, rye, and barley, causes a reactive immune response resulting in GI symptoms in people with celiac disease. People with celiac disease and gluten intolerance can also experience brain and neurologic symptoms ranging from walking problems, peripheral neuropathy, depression, headache, and muscle inflammation, reinforcing the connection between diet, inflammation, and brain health. Treatment includes adhering to a strict gluten-free diet (eliminating wheat, rye, oats, and barley, including the flour used in baked goods and pasta).

There is, however, no established connection between gluten and PD except one case report that describes a person with celiac disease and improved parkinsonian movement symptoms after adopting a three-month gluten-free diet to treat confirmed celiac disease. SPECT[4] brain imaging did confirm low dopamine levels in the basal ganglia both before and after dietary treatment, but no change in dopamine nerve cell levels after the change in diet. Gluten does cause inflammation in patients with celiac disease, and brain immune-mediated inflammation is measured in brain autopsies of people with celiac disease and neurologic symptoms. In the published case noted, both chronic inflammation and related nutritional deficiencies from poor absorption of nutrients can cause enough stress to exacerbate motor symptoms. How these findings relate to people without celiac is unclear as no association is made between gluten and PD-related nerve changes.

Ketogenic diet. This high fat, low carbohydrate diet has long been known to improve seizure control in children with medicine refractory epilepsy. When

---

[4] Single-photon emission computed tomography (SPECT) is a nuclear medicine imaging technique.

glucose levels are low, ketones are produced from fatty acids in the liver. Ketones are the most efficient source of energy for brain cells and are actively studied for their neuroprotective effects. Animal studies show that ketone bodies can prevent the damage inflicted by 1-methyl-4-phenyl-1,2,3,6-tetrahydropyridine (MPTP) on dopamine nerve cells and can prevent the damage to mitochondria from pesticides (rotenone) that cause parkinsonism in animals. There is only one small study in PD with improved movement scores noted in five of seven people. This study, however, did not control for the placebo effect. The ketogenic diet can elevate cholesterol and exacerbate osteoporosis. Coconut oil, metabolized to ketones, is also under study with mixed results for diseases such as epilepsy, Alzheimer's disease, and PD.

Organic foods. Exposure to pesticides is the strongest link between the environment and PD. Eating organic foods can reduce ingestion of pesticides, but organic produce is expensive. Be sure to wash all produce in warm water with mild soap if organic foods are not an option. Foods with thick skins or peels have lower pesticide levels. The Dirty Dozen and Clean Fifteen are lists of foods (available on the Internet) with higher and lower pesticide exposure, respectively, to help you choose which foods to eat organic.

STRESS MANAGEMENT

Stress is a major contributor to chronic illness. In fact, over 70% of illness is caused or worsened by stress. I have interviewed countless people who describe their first PD symptoms beginning at the time of a significant life stress. Sometimes the symptoms disappear only to return later in life. Think about how stress changes your symptoms. It is not uncommon for the following movement symptoms to worsen abruptly in the face of stress:

- Tremor
- Dystonia
- Dyskinesia
- Freezing of gait (FoG)

Stress can also worsen non-motor symptoms such as pain, depression, anxiety, sleep, and digestion. Most important, stress can have a long-term impact as it will influence your emotional outlook, motivation, sense of hopefulness, ability to problem-solve and make positive lifestyle choices, and your resiliency to overcome obstacles in life.

Some stress in life can be avoided. Other types of stress cannot. Fortunately, the negative impact of stress on health and disease is not simply related to whether you have stress in your life but, more importantly, how you respond to that stress. Taking action and feeling a sense of control are important first steps.

One way to reduce stress is to simplify your life. Easier said than done, given the growing number of tasks and activities that fill up your busy day—work, children, home, mortgage, medical care, caregiving, exercise, the list goes on.

But there are some things you can do to simplify life and reduce the stress that comes with multitasking and overextending yourself. Simplifying your life does not necessarily mean living without or on less. It means living thoughtfully and deliberately by exploring what is important to your life, what gives meaning to you, and what robs you of your energy and well-being.

An important first step is to prioritize your activities and tasks to include those that are necessary and important to you. Seek help when you need it, delegate when possible, and learn to say no if you are overwhelmed. Plan for the worse and celebrate the best. Having a plan in place for difficult times, changes in independence, or medical illness will help you maintain a sense of control and influence over the direction of change.

Mind-body techniques can help you gain control over the moment, reduce the impact of stress, increase your emotional and physical resiliency, and help you see positive solutions to your problems. These techniques influence the autonomic nervous system to reduce the sympathetic fight-or-flight response and engage the parasympathetic or relaxation response.

The following table is a review of specific bodily functions and symptoms regulated by these two important branches of the autonomic nervous system. The symptoms in **bold** represent unique symptoms that are both under involuntary neurologic control and voluntary control.

PHYSIOLOGIC RESPONSE	
SYMPATHETIC "FIGHT OR FLIGHT"	PARASYMPATHETIC "RECOVERY AND RELAXATION"
Thoughts and feelings of distress	**Thoughts and feelings of well-being**
Hypervigilance and anxiety	Reduced anxiety
Dilated pupils	Smaller pupils
Sweating	
Rapid breathing	**Slow, rhythmic breathing**
Racing heart	Reduced heart rate
Increased blood pressure	Reduced blood pressure
Shunt of blood from digestive organs to muscle	Improved digestion
Increased muscle tension	**Reduced muscle tension**

Mind-body techniques focus on the voluntary control of these symptoms, in effect creating behavioral and neurologic feedback loops that will alter involuntary control and the activity of these nerve circuits! It is no surprise that mind-body techniques focus on body activities that are regulated by these pathways but can also be easily and voluntarily changed. For instance:

- *Breathing:* meditation and therapeutic yoga
- *Emotional and cognitive thoughts:* guided imagery, meditation, cognitive therapies, hypnosis, positive affirmation, and prayer
- *Muscle control and tension:* massage and yoga

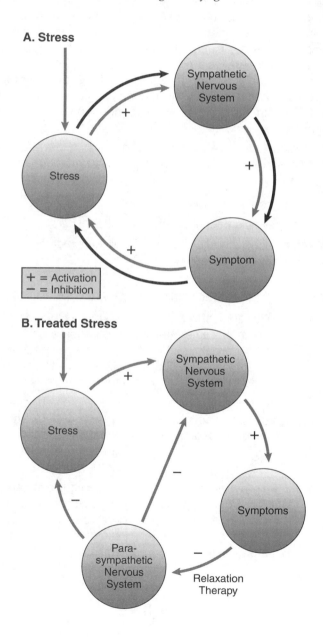

CLINICAL PEARL: CHANGE YOUR STRESS AND YOUR BODY

Three activities, e.g., breathing, muscle tension, and cognitive thoughts, mimic how the sympathetic (stress) and parasympathetic (relaxation) system influence body function. The exercise that follows illustrates the concept of the neurologic feedback loop. The symptoms experienced during this exercise influence nerve connections that "feed back" to the brain to drive yet more symptoms. Intentionally shifting your thoughts, pattern of breathing, or muscle tension can break that cycle by further engaging the parasympathetic response. This simple exercise is the foundation by which many stress management techniques work.

Exercise: Sit quietly, close your eyes, and spend a few minutes performing each of the activities described. Pay attention to how you feel as you do so.

- Does one feel better than the other?
- Which activity is easier for you to control?
- Which activity or body function do you feel you can work with in your daily practice to help you relax?

ACTIVITY	SYMPATHETIC CONTROL	PARASYMPATHETIC CONTROL
Breathing	Take rapid, short, and irregular breaths. Breathe shallow breaths, taking air into your throat but not deep into the lungs.	Take slow, big, deep, and regular breaths. Bring each breath deep into your lungs. Breathe in and exhale slowly.
Muscle tension	Tighten and clench your neck, shoulders, and fists for 5 seconds.	Settle into your chair and relax your neck and shoulders. Rest your hands on your lap and close your eyes.
Thoughts	Take a moment and think about all of the things you need to do today and that you may not get done.	Close your eyes and think of a favorite place or time, such as the beach or vacation, or the joy and smile of a child.

(continued)

CLINICAL PEARL (*continued*)

Set aside time, even just five minutes, to intentionally relax. Make this part of your routine. Over time you will learn to listen to your body, recognize your own symptoms of stress, and minimize its effect. The stress and anxiety inventory in Part V, Personalize Your Care, will help increase your awareness of stress and its impact on you.

Mindfulness

Mindfulness is a powerful technique of intentionally bringing awareness, without judgment, to the present moment. This state of awareness joins mind, emotions, senses, and body together as a whole, allowing you to be fully present and engaged in the "now." Mindfulness coupled with the practice of non-judgment—or the ability to simply notice a symptom, a feeling, a sensation, or an experience without attaching a label or reaction—brings awareness to the thoughts and ideas that can influence how you *react and feel*.

This technique is particularly powerful for those of you living with PD since you can influence how you feel and respond to any difficulties when they occur. For instance, you may have distressing thoughts about your tremor. The more you attach these thoughts to your tremor, the greater your negative reaction to tremor in the moment. Your thoughts spiral downward . . . more distress creates more tremor creates more distress. Awareness without judgment allows you to choose an alternative response. For example, when tremor increases you now have one of two choices: to react or to respond. These choices at first glance seem very similar but they are indeed very different in mindset and outcome.

React. By reacting to tremor you are giving control to the spontaneous thoughts and feelings that affect how you feel. Your spontaneous thoughts are unique to you but often include judgments: *"Tremor is ruining my life. My disease is getting worse. I must fix this or stop this now. If only I didn't have tremor everything would be fine. What if someone sees my tremor?"* These automatic and reactive thoughts lead to a snowball effect, further worsening stress and increasing tremor.

Respond. By responding to tremor you are no longer reacting but instead observing and choosing how to respond. *"I recognize this feeling. This problem will pass. I will not let this get the best of me. I will sit for a few minutes to let this pass. I have experienced tremor before and I will get through this. This is just a moment; it is not my future, and tomorrow is another day. The tremor is in my hands but is not me."* By choosing your response you gain a sense of control and change the very relationship you have to your disease or symptom.

This does not mean that you have given in to your symptoms or enjoy the fact that you have PD, but it does reduce the downward spiral that can occur when symptoms are most noticeable. By strengthening the connection between mind-body you gain a better understanding of your integration of thoughts, emotions, sensations, and physical body and how each of these areas affects you. There are many other ways that mindfulness can help a person or caregiver living with PD.

Appreciate the simple moments. When added together, the otherwise overlooked comes into focus to weave the rich tapestry that is life. When was the last time you truly "felt" the smile of a loved one or "saw" the delicate nature of dew drops hanging on the leaves at dawn or the poetic beauty of the sunset. PD does not "steal" these moments of richness.

Attention to the moment brings attention to the now, to the subtle, to the important. We are living now. Not in the regrets or losses of the past or fear of the future. We often spend so much time judging or mourning the past and planning or worrying about the future that we are not present and fully appreciative of the present moment. Bringing awareness to the present is a helpful way to manage change, future worries, uncertainty, and feelings of lack of control after diagnosis.

Live in the present to expand the power of possibility. As you choose how to respond to problems in the present you intentionally impact the present with each step (moment) guiding the next.

Stress causes illness. Stress increases PD symptoms especially tremor, dyskinesia, and freezing of gait. Stress negatively affects your brain even at the cellular and genetic level. Mindfulness reduces the physiologic impact of stress on your body and mind, improving how you feel.

Mindfulness "rewires" the brain. This is a process called neuroplasticity. Mindfulness-based meditation enhances frontal lobe activity in regions important for cognitive and emotional processing and reduces activity in the amygdala, a brain region that is driven by distress. Mindfulness meditation, when used by people with PD, has been shown to cause changes in brain volume in the amygdala and hippocampus (important structures for mediating stress and memory, respectively). Together these changes enhance emotional resiliency and constructive reasoning, attributes so important to living well with a chronic condition.

Mindfulness is free, portable, and available to everyone. It can be an informal practice in which daily experiences are used as an opportunity to be present. The next time you awaken to a sunrise, walk in the park, hear the laughter of a child, are stuck in traffic, or feel the shaking in your hand, you can practice mindfulness.

Mindfulness is also practiced as a formal exercise with meditation. One way to practice mindfulness meditation is to sit quietly and calmly but with attention and awareness. Bringing your attention to your breathing is one way to bring focus to the moment. During this time you will simply observe your thoughts, feelings, sensations. and perceptions and let them pass without judging them, labeling them, or controlling them. Meditation is a practice and as such the benefits will improve with time. Mindfulness meditation is not without risk. Individuals with psychotic disorders, significant depression, or post-traumatic stress disorder should meditate under the care of a mental health professional.

> *Sit*
> *for a moment.*
>
> *Close your eyes.*
> *What is in front of you,*
> *surrounds you.*
>
> *Listen,*
> *feel.*
> *Take in the unexpected!*
>
> *Open your eyes.*
> *Move forward*
> *in stillness.*
>
> *All this*
> *in a moment.*
>
> *—Monique L. Giroux, MD*

With practice, mindfulness can also be experienced during everyday activities as simple as eating. Mindful eating is not a diet. Mindful eating is about experiencing your food—the pleasure, taste, texture, color, source, and abundance. Mindful eating connects your body's needs to the experience while eating. Mindful eating also extends to the preparation and even gratitude for the many steps—the people, farmers, hard work, and organizations—that bring food to the table. Think about your last few meals:

- Did your meal, mealtime, and meal companions have your full attention?
- Did you taste your food?
- Did you take the time to eat?

If you answered no to any of these questions, you may not be getting the benefits that accompany healthful eating. The following suggestions will enhance the way food can heal.

- Set the time aside to be present during a meal or snack.
- Reflect on the healing and nourishing power of food.
- Feel positive about the healthy food choices that you make to further encourage these choices and strengthen the healing effect.
- Taste, feel, and see your food. Be especially sure to taste, feel, and see your food when you indulge in a pleasurable snack.
- Turn off the TV, computer, and other distractions so that you can be present with your dinner companion(s) during meals.
- Think with gratitude about how your food got to you and was prepared.

CLINICAL PEARL: STRENGTHENING THE MIND-BODY CONNECTION IS AS SIMPLE AS POSTURE

Postural changes with PD and age are common. These postural changes can have far-reaching effects beyond the spine. There is a tendency toward forward flexion at the hips, waist, shoulders, and neck. Flexed posture results in other physical changes. Center of gravity shifts ahead of the feet. Knees and hips bend to prevent from falling forward. Steps become smaller and walking is slower. Stamina can be reduced as gait biomechanics become less efficient. Bent posture can also impact breathing by constricting lung expansion. Speech becomes softer and swallowing more difficulty.

The effects of posture are more than physical. Posture reflects how you feel and changes how you feel. Posture is perhaps one of the most impactful body positions when it comes to mind-body connection. Researchers evaluated the effect of sitting slouched vs. erect in a chair. This simple intervention had some dramatic results.

Body Influencing Mind

- Erect posture is associated with improved self-confidence and positive thoughts about self.
- Erect posture improves motor and cognitive reaction time or speed.
- Slumped posture changes perceptions of stress and sense of helplessness.
- Posing in a "high powerful" way increases testosterone, cortisol, and risk-taking behavior.

Mind Influencing Body

- Depression and sadness tend to increase slumped posture and even walking by influencing both speed and arm swing.

Two important concepts can be derived from these observations:

1. The mind-body connection is influenced in both directions.
2. Simple changes can make a difference.

(continued)

CLINICAL PEARL (continued)

Next Steps

- Take a moment to be aware of your posture. Use a mirror to identify changes that may occur.
- See your physical therapist to get started with posture exercises early in the disease process.
- Focus on programs that place emphasis on posture, mindfulness, body awareness, and creative expression such as yoga, dance, and Feldenkrais Method®.
- Expand your chest, "tune into the breath," and invoke a sense of calm.
- Use your posture to affect how you feel. Sit and stand tall when you feel sad or less energetic and confident.

TELEVISION

Television, smartphone, and computers are changing the way we live, giving us access to new ideas, information, and resources. If left unchecked, time spent watching television and/or on a smartphone or computer has the potential of taking us away from the attention and time needed to improve our physical and emotional well-being. Excessive time spent watching TV or using the computer leads to eye strain, sleepiness, and most important of all robs you from time otherwise spent engaged in life activities, social engagements, outdoor pursuits, and nature activities.

Although there are no objective studies, TV and device use appears to be greater in people with PD. Reasons are many and could be related to late-night sleep problems, social isolation, limited physical activity, or impulsivity issues. Take note of the number of hours you use the computer or TV each day and aim to replace some of this time with an alternative activity such as reading, walking, creative hobbies, cooking, or socializing.

SLEEP

Sleep is often fragmented by poor quality, defined by frequent and early awakening. Depression, anxiety tremor, pain, dystonia, frequent urination, physical discomfort, and trouble turning in bed are just a few of the PD-related problems that can impair sleep. Sleep is often affected by medication wearing off and the return of motor and non-motor symptoms at night, since there is often a long duration of time between doses. Non-motor off symptoms that can interrupt sleep are drenching sweats, restless legs syndrome, and anxiety. Motor off symptoms that commonly interrupt sleep are tremor, dystonia, and cramping (especially in the legs and feet). Other sleep related problems more common in PD are sleep apnea and REM sleep disorder.[5]

Daytime motor symptoms, fatigue, depression, and confusion are often worse when sleep is poor. Fortunately there are many things you can do to sleep better. Some of these steps are reviewed in Chapter 13.

PASSION AND CREATIVITY

Goal-driven behavior and creativity is mediated by dopamine. In fact, treatment of PD movement symptoms with dopaminergic medicines may be associated with an increase in creative pursuits. This is an important therapeutic opportunity worthy of exploration. There are many benefits that can be obtained through creative expression including:

- Personal empowerment that comes with the mastering of a new activity
- Enhanced neuroplasticity associated with activities that are new, complex, emotionally meaningful, social, and involve sensory-motor-emotional integration
- Expression of sense of self not defined by disease
- Improved social contact
- Reduced stress, loneliness, and depression
- Improved life engagement, hope, and participation in other healthful lifestyle activities
- Participation in creative arts, which leads to new ways of self-expression, creative ideas and ways of seeing and overcoming obstacles
- Reduced cognitive decline, risk, and progression of dementia

Reflect on your day-to-day activities. Are you a creature of habit? Are there opportunities to try new things and/or diversify your extracurricular activities?

In this chapter, you have learned about the importance of your lifestyle and lifestyle choices to your disease, overall health, and emotional well-being. The next section reviews specific integrative therapies. Many of these therapies support the positive lifestyle choices so important to living your best with PD.

---

[5] REM sleep disorder describes a change during dream stage of sleep. In this condition, muscle tone that is usually lost in dream sleep is maintained. Dreams are more vivid and assertive and, coupled with retained muscle tone, can lead to screaming, punching, and physical "acting out dreams."

References

Weight Management

Horstmann, A. 2011. "Obesity-related differences between women and men in brain structure and goal-directed behavior." *Frontiers in Human Neuroscience* 5: 58.

Kashihara, K. 2006. "Weight loss in Parkinson's disease." *Journal of Neurology* 253: S7 VII38–41.

Kurth, F., et al. 2013. "Relationships between gray matter, body mass index, and waist circumference in healthy adults." *Human Brain Mapping* 34: 1737–46.

Maswood, N., et al. 2004. "Caloric restriction increases neurotrophic factor levels and attenuates neurochemical and behavioral deficits in a primate model of Parkinson's disease." *Proceedings of the National Academy of Science* 101: 18171–176.

Mills, K. A., et al. 2012. "Weight change after globus pallidus internus or subthalamic nucleus deep brain stimulation in Parkinson's disease and dystonia." *Stereotactic Functional Neurosurgery* 90: 386–93.

Novakova, L., et al. 2011. "Hormonal regulators of food intake and weight gain in Parkinson's disease after subthalamic nucleus stimulation." *Neuroendocrinology Letters* 32: 437–41.

Srivastava, S., and M. C. Haigis. 2011. "Role of sirtuins and calorie restriction in neuroprotection: implications in Alzheimer's and Parkinson's diseases." *Current Pharmaceutical Design* 17: 3418–33.

Wank, G. J. 2001. "Brain dopamine and obesity." *Lancet* 357: 354–57.

Tobacco and Alcohol Use

Benedetti, M. B., et al. 2000. "Smoking, alcohol, and coffee consumption preceding Parkinson's disease: A case control study." *Neurology* 55: 1350–58.

Chen et al. "Does alcohol consumption reduce the risk of Parkinson's?" American Neurological Association (ANA) 136th Annual Meeting: Poster S208. Presented September 25, 2011.

Guo, X., et al. 2012. "Alcohol Consumption, Types of Alcohol, and Parkinson's disease." *PLoS One* 8: e66452.

Exercise

Ahlskog, J. E. 2011. "Does vigorous exercise have a neuroprotective effect in Parkinson disease?" *Neurology* 77: 288–94.

Allen, N. E. 2010. "The effects of an exercise program on fall risk factors in people with Parkinson's disease: A randomized controlled trial." *Movement Disorders* 25: 1217–25.

Ashburn, A., et al. 2007. "A randomized controlled trial of a home-based exercise programme to reduce the risk of falling among people with Parkinson's disease." *Journal of Neurology, Neurosurgery, and Psychiatry* 78: 678–84.

Canning, C. G. 1997. "Parkinson's disease: An investigation of exercise capacity, respiratory function, and gait." *Archive of Physical Medicine and Rehabilitation* 78: 199–207.

———. 2014. "Exercise for falls prevention in Parkinson disease: A randomized controlled trial. *Neurology* 84: 304–31.

Chen, H., et al. 2005. "Physical activity and the risk of Parkinson's." *Neurology* 64: 664–69.

De Dreu, M. J. 2012. "Rehabilitation, exercise therapy, and music in patients with Parkinson's disease: a meta-analysis of the effects of music-based movement therapy on walking ability, balance, and quality of life." *Parkinsonism and Related Disorders* 18S: 114–19.

Dibble, L. E., et al. 2009. "High-intensity eccentric resistance training decreases bradykinesia and improves quality of life in persons with Parkinson's disease: A preliminary study." *Parkinson's and Related Disorders* 15: 752–57.

———. 2009. "The effects of exercise on balance in persons with Parkinson's disease: A systematic review across the disability spectrum." *Journal of Neurologic Physical Therapy* 33: 14–26.

Fietzek, U. M. 2014. "Randomized cross-over trial to investigate the efficacy of a two-week physiotherapy programme with repetitive exercises of cueing to reduce the severity of freezing of gait in patients with Parkinson's disease." *Clinical Rehabilitation.* http://m.cre.sagepub.com/content/28/9/902

Fisher, B. E., et al. 2013. "Treadmill exercise elevates striatal dopamine D2 receptor binding potential in patients with early Parkinson's disease." *Neuroreport* 24: 509–14.

Frazzitta, G., et al. 2012. "Rehabilitation improves dyskinesias in Parkinsonian patients: A pilot study comparing two different rehabilitative treatments." *Neuro-Rehabilitation* 30: 295–301.

Goodwin, V. A., et al. 2008. "The effectiveness of exercise intervention for people with Parkinson's disease: A systemic meta-analysis." *Movement Disorders* 23: 631–40.

Hakney, M. E., et al. 2009. "Effects of dance on movement control in Parkinson's disease: A comparison of Argentine tango and American ballroom." *Journal of Rehabilitation Medicine* 41: 475–81.

Kuroda, K., et al. 1992. "Effect of physical exercise on mortality in patients with Parkinson's disease." *Acta Neurologica Scandinavica* 86: 55–59.

Petzinger, G. M., et al. 2013. "Exercise-enhanced neuroplasticity targeting motor and cognitive circuitry in Parkinson's disease." *Lancet Neurology* 12: 716–26.

Qi, G., et al. 2014. "Effects of Tai Chi on balance and fall prevention in Parkinson's disease: A randomized controlled trial." *Clinical Rehabilitation* 28: 748–53.

Ridgel, A. L., et al. 2009. "Forced, not voluntary, exercise improves motor function in Parkinson's disease patients." *Neurorehabilitation and Neural Repair* 23: 600–8.

Sääksjärvi, K., et al. 2014. "Reduced risk of Parkinson's disease associated with lower body mass index and heavy leisure-time physical activity." *European Journal of Epidemiology* 29: 285–92.

Schenkman, M., et al. 1998. "Exercise to improve spinal flexibility and function for people with Parkinson's disease: A randomized, controlled trial." *Journal of the American Geriatrics Society* 46: 1207–16.

Sharma, N. K., et al. 2015. "A randomized controlled pilot study of the therapeutic effects of yoga in people with Parkinson's disease." *International Yoga Journal* 8: 74–79.

Shulman, L. M., et al. 2013. "Randomized clinical trial of 3 types of physical exercise for patients with Parkinson disease." *JAMA Neurology* 70: 183–90.

Tillerson, J. L., et al. 2003. "Exercise induces behavioral recovery and attenuates neurochemical deficits in rodent models of Parkinson's disease." *Neuroscience* 119: 899–911.

Yang, F., et al. 2015. "Physical activity and risk of Parkinson's disease in the Swedish National March Cohort." *Brain* 138: 269–75.

Nutrition

Alcaly, et al. 2012. "The Association between Mediterranean Diet Adherence and Parkinson's disease." *Movement Disorders* 27: 771–74.

Cereda, E., et al. 2013. "Diabetes and risk of Parkinson's disease." *Movement Disorders* 28: 257–61.

Chen, H., et al. 2007. "Consumption of dairy products and risk of Parkinson's disease." *American Journal of Epidemiology* 165: 998–1006.

DiLazzaro, V., et al. 2014. "Dramatic improvement of parkinsonian symptoms after gluten-free diet introduction in a patient with silent celiac disease." *Journal of Neurology* 261: 443–45.

Gao, X., et al. 2007. "Prospective study of dietary pattern and risk of Parkinson disease." *American Journal of Clinical Nutrition* 86: 1486–94.

Mena, I., and C. Cotzias. 1975. "Protein intake and treatment of Parkinson's disease with levodopa." *New England Journal of Medicine* 292: 181–84.

Pottala, J. V. 2014. "Higher RBC EPA + DHA corresponds with larger total brain and hippocampal volumes: WHIMS-MRI Study." *Neurology* 82: 435–42.

Prediger, R. D. 2010. "Effects of caffeine in Parkinson's disease: from neuroprotection to the management of motor and non-motor symptoms." *Journal of Alzheimer's Disease* S1: S205.

Silva, D., et al. 2008. "Depression in Parkinson's disease: A double-blind, randomized, placebo-controlled pilot study of omega-3 fatty-acid supplementation." *Journal of Affective Disorders* 111: 351–59.

Simopoulus, A. P. 2002. "The importance of the ratio of omega-6/omega-3 essential fatty acids." *Biomed Pharmacotherapy* 56: 3365–79.

Prakash, K. M., and E. K. Tan. 2011. "Clinical evidence linking coffee and tea intake with Parkinson's disease." *Basal Ganglia* 1: 127–30.

Stafstrom, C. E., and J. M. Rho. 2012. "The ketogenic diet as a treatment paradigm for diverse neurological disorders." *Frontiers in Pharmacology* 3: 59.

Turner, B. L., and A. L. Thompson. 2013. "Beyond the Paleolithic prescription: incorporating diversity and flexibility in the study of human diet evolution." *Nutrition Review* 71: 501–510.

Vanitallie, T. B., et al. 2005. "Treatment of Parkinson disease with diet-induced hyperketonemia: a feasibility study." *Neurology* 64: 728–30.

Stress Management

Brinol, P., et al. 2009. "Body posture effects on self-evaluation: A self-validation approach." *European Journal of Social Psychology* 39: 1053–64.

Carney, D. R., et al. 2010. "Power posing: Brief nonverbal displays affect neuroendocrine levels and risk tolerance." *Psychological Science* 21: 1363–68.

Fitzpatrick, L., 2010. "A qualitative analysis of mindfulness-based cognitive therapy (MBCT) in Parkinson's disease." *Psychology and Psychotherapy: Theory, Research, and Practice* 83: 179–92.

Johannes, M., et al. 2009. "Embodiment of sadness and depression: Gait patterns associated with dysphoric mood." *Psychosomatic Medicine* 71: 580–87.

Pickut, B. A., et al. 2013. "Mindfulness-based intervention in Parkinson's disease leads to structural changes on MRI: a randomized controlled trial." *Clinical Neurology and Neurosurgery* 115: 2419–25.

Riskind, J. H., and C. C. Gotay. 1982. "Physical posture: Could it have regulatory or feedback effects on motivation and emotion? *Motivation and Emotion* 6: n273–98.

Schlesinger, I., et al. 2004. "Parkinson's disease tremor is diminished with relaxation guided imagery." *Movement Disorders* 24: 2059–62.

Passion and Creativity

Cohen, D. 2006. "Research on creativity and aging: The positive impact of the arts on health and illness." *Generations* 30: 7–15.

Inzelberg, R. 2013. "The awakening of artistic creativity and Parkinson's disease." *Behavioral Neuroscience* 127: 256–61.

Verghese, J., et al. 2003. "Leisure activities and the risk of dementia in the elderly." *New England Journal of Medicine* 348: 2508–16.

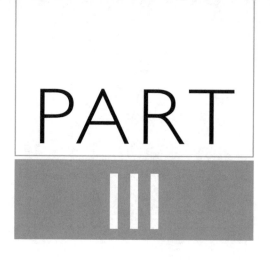

Integrative Therapies

Just what therapies are available, what do they do, and which one is right for you? For some of you, this is the section for which you have been waiting. Here you will learn about the more common therapies available to you using a modification of the classification set forth by the National Center for Complementary and Integrative Health biological therapies, body therapies, mind-body therapies, energy and sensory therapies, and whole system approaches. A description of each therapy, how it is proposed to work, its use in Parkinson's, and precautions will be presented. If available, guidance to help you find a qualified practitioner or treatment, including professional training or certification, is included.

An "Interview with the Expert" is included for many of these therapies so that you can learn from the real-life experience of practitioners treating people with Parkinson's disease.

CHAPTER

6

Biological Therapies

Biological therapies include plant-derived chemicals and products, vitamins, and supplements. Biological therapies are used to promote cell health and healing, control symptoms, and improve emotional well-being. Biological therapies are organized by their proposed mechanism of action as follows (some supplements fall into multiple categories):

- *Vitamins and Minerals:* micronutrients and macronutrients required in small and trace quantities to orchestrate a range of physiological and cell functions

- *Antioxidants:* agents that reduce the cell-damaging effect of oxidative stress, a by-product of cell metabolism and proposed cause of nerve cell death in Parkinson's disease (PD)

- *Anti-inflammatories:* agents that reduce cellular inflammation, a proposed cause of nerve cell death in PD

- *Bioenergetics:* agents that enhance cell energy production or serve as a brain or muscle energy source

- *Immunomodulators:* agents that interact with our brain's immune health and circadian body rhythms or control

- *Neurochemicals and Amino Acids:* agents that are precursors to neurotransmitters used by nerve cells

- *Botanicals:* chemical derivatives or plant-based agents used for their medicinal properties, including some that contain levodopa or dopamine

VITAMINS AND MINERALS

Vitamins are complex organic chemicals (i.e., can be broken down by chemical reaction) and minerals are inorganic compounds (i.e., cannot be broken down by chemical reaction) not produced by the body but needed in small amounts for normal cell growth and development.

There are two types of vitamins: fat soluble and water soluble. Water soluble vitamins are not stored in body tissue, so excess vitamins are eliminated in the urine or stool. Fat soluble vitamins are stored in fat (as are other fat soluble chemicals and toxins). Excess intake of these vitamins can lead to toxic levels.

- Fat soluble vitamins include vitamins A, D, K, and E.
- Water soluble vitamins include vitamin C and B (B12, B6, thiamine, folate).

Minerals can be separated into two categories—micronutrients and macronutrients—based on the amount needed by the body.

- Micronutrients include iron, copper, selenium, and zinc.
- Macronutrients include calcium, potassium, magnesium, and sodium.

Select vitamins and minerals of interest to PD are reviewed in the following pages.

CLINICAL PEARL: SUPPLEMENT SAFETY

Tips to follow when shopping for vitamins and supplements

The Food and Drug Administration (FDA) regulates the safe and accurate use of prescription medicines but does not regulate vitamins and supplements in the same way. At present it is the manufacturer's responsibility to ensure that its product is safe, pure, free of contaminants, and accurate as to the potency or dosage.

This, of course, requires that manufacturers "police themselves." This requires you, as the consumer, to take extra precautionary steps. The following tips can help you when you purchase vitamins and supplements:

(continued)

CLINICAL PEARL (*continued*)

- Although taking a pill is easier, remember in many cases the best defense and best results occur when nutritional substances, including vitamins and minerals, come from a healthy diet, not a pill.

- Beware of marketing hype. If claims are too good to be true, they probably are. Just because something is described as "natural" or an "herb" does not mean it is safe, effective, or free of contamination.

- Supplements and vitamins can interact with your current prescription medicines. For example, St. John's wort, fish oil, garlic, vitamin E, and ginkgo biloba are examples of supplements used by some PD patients that can interact with warfarin to increase bleeding. St. John's wort cannot be used with a common PD medicine rasagiline (Azilect®).

- Be sure that the label reflects what is needed. If you are purchasing fish oil based on the benefit of DHA and EPA, are the amounts of these compounds measured and listed on the product label?

- Look for products that are tested for purity, potency, and bioavailability (i.e., how it is absorbed by the body) by an independent laboratory. This ensures accurate and unbiased reporting. Search for products that carry United States Pharmacopeia (USP) verification. The U.S. Pharmacopeial Convention is a scientific nonprofit organization that sets standards for the identity, strength, quality, and purity of medicines, food ingredients, and dietary supplements manufactured, distributed, and consumed worldwide. This independent laboratory tests the purity, potency, and bioavailability of products—in effect, ensuring what is on the bottle label is indeed what is contained in the pill or supplement. Otherwise the actual purity and strength of the substance may not be the same as the bottle label. Consumer Lab is another good resource that tests different brand names and can give you the same information.

Website Resources

Food and Drug Administration, www.fda.gov/Food

Consumer Lab, www.consumerlab.com

U.S. Pharmacopeial Convention, www.usp.org

Calcium
Description and Mechanism of Action
Calcium is a mineral important for bone health and regulation of cell and nerve activity. Calcium strengthens bone by incorporating into the bone matrix to harden bone. In fact, 99% of calcium is stored in bone and teeth. Calcium in the form of calcium carbonate buffers the pH of stomach acid. Calcium also interacts with ion channels located on nerve and muscle cell membranes to regulate nerve activity, smooth muscle (blood vessels, heart, and gastrointestinal tract), and skeletal muscle contraction.

Use in Parkinson's
Calcium is used to ensure strong bones and thereby reduce the risk of osteoporosis or bone thinning and fractures from falls. The risk of osteoporosis and risk of fracture from falls increases with age. Together, calcium and vitamin D may reduce the risk of falls through blood pressure control and reduced postural sway. Calcium is sometimes used for headache, muscle cramping, and symptoms of acid reflux.

Precautions
A meta-analysis of 15 studies and over 8,000 people, analyzing the effect of daily calcium supplement doses greater than 500 mg in people over the age of 40, has revealed a 30% increased risk of heart attack. The authors of this study state that "treatment of 1,000 people with calcium for five years would cause an additional 14 myocardial infarctions, 10 strokes, and 13 deaths, and prevent 26 fractures."

Guidance
Talk to your doctor about your calcium intake and avoid high dose calcium supplementation unless recommended by your doctor. Most men need 1,000 to 1,200 mg of calcium daily and women need about 1,200 mg daily. Included in this amount is the calcium you get from foods, which should be used in estimating your total dose of supplement. Be sure to add the extra calcium you are getting from a multiple vitamin if you are taking one. Only 500 mg of calcium in tablet form can be absorbed at one time.

Calcium carbonate is cheaper but best absorbed after meals or with orange juice, since it must be dissolved by stomach acid. Calcium carbonate pills are larger and hard for some people with Parkinson's to swallow.

Calcium citrate does not require stomach acid to dissolve; pills are smaller in size but more expensive.

Oxalic acid binds with calcium to block its absorption by the gastrointestinal tract. Spinach, chard, and beet greens are high in this compound and will therefore reduce calcium absorption if eaten at the same time you take a calcium pill.

Calcium-rich foods include:

- Milk, 1 cup: 300 mg
- Yogurt, 1 cup: 350 mg
- Cheese, 1 oz.: 150–200 mg
- Salmon, 3 oz.: 200 mg (more with bones)
- Tofu, 3 oz.: 150 mg
- Nondairy foods such as soy milk, almond milk, and orange juice fortified with calcium (read your labels)

Iron and Manganese
Description and Mechanism of Action
Iron and manganese are minerals found in all cells. Iron is needed for cell growth and many biochemical reactions. It is an important part of hemoglobin, a protein in blood that carries and transfers oxygen from the blood to tissue. Manganese is also important to biochemical reactions as well as bone and connective tissue health.

Use in Parkinson's
Low levels of iron can cause or exacerbate restless legs syndrome, a problem associated with PD, causing nighttime sleep discomfort and daytime fatigue. Low iron levels can also cause anemia. Although anemia is not related to PD, it can worsen PD symptoms of fatigue and dizziness.

The relationship between iron and PD is complex. Iron levels are high in the brain tissue of people with PD, suggesting this mineral plays a role in cellular destruction. Recent studies measuring iron in the blood suggest that low and not high blood levels of iron increase the risk of PD.

Manganese is an important mineral for enzymatic processing, including the production of antioxidants in the body. Manganese toxicity is not common but can cause atypical parkinsonism. This form of parkinsonism is not caused by dopamine nerve cell damage in the substantia nigra, as seen in PD. Rapid progression, early balance and walking problems, significant psychiatric symptoms, and lack of response to levodopa differentiate manganese parkinsonism from PD. Manganese is found in the soil and in many foods, and may be found in high levels in some supplements such as chondroitin and glucosamine used for joint health.

Precautions
Iron contributes to oxidative stress and may play a role in abnormal protein aggregation (alpha synuclein) in the brain. Excessive iron is deposited in organs and can cause damage to skin, bone, and liver. Because of these potential toxic effects, supplementation is not recommended unless advised and monitored by your doctor or health care provider.

Iron pills should not be taken with levodopa since iron can reduce the absorption of this important medicine.

Guidance

Most men and postmenopausal women do not need iron supplementation. Iron deficiency can be diagnosed with a simple blood test, which is a helpful guide for treatment.

Foods high in iron include:

- Meat
- Seafood
- Beans
- Green leafy vegetables
- Nuts
- Apricots, peaches, and prunes

Note: Iron from non-meat sources is poorly absorbed. Oxalic acid found in beans and spinach will decrease iron absorption. Vitamin C increases iron absorption.

Manganese is an antioxidant that has health benefits. Obtain manganese from food instead of supplements to avoid toxic levels.

Foods high in manganese include:

- Meat
- Green leafy vegetables especially spinach and kale
- Hazel nuts and pumpkin seeds
- Beans
- Soy

Magnesium

Description and Mechanism of Action

Magnesium is a macronutrient needed for many cellular activities including bone health, muscle, and nerve control. Magnesium regulates cellular physiology with particular effects on muscle and nerve cells. Magnesium can reduce nerve cell hyper-excitability and muscular contraction.

Use in Parkinson's

Magnesium is commonly prescribed for muscle spasm and nighttime muscle cramps. It is also a laxative so is often used in low doses for constipation.

Precautions

Magnesium can be toxic at very high levels or if you have kidney disease.

Guidance

Magnesium citrate and oxide can help constipation but can also cause diarrhea at high doses. Magnesium glycinate has a lower risk of diarrhea. It is best to avoid doses over 400 mg unless prescribed by your healthcare provider.

The DASH[1] diet for high blood pressure is particularly high in magnesium.

Magnesium-rich foods include:

- Foods high in fiber are often high in magnesium
- Beans, seeds, and nuts (especially almonds)
- Broccoli, squash, green leafy vegetables
- Whole grains

Selenium and Zinc

Description and Mechanism of Action

Selenium and zinc are trace elements found in foods and have many chemical roles, including immune health, wound healing, DNA production, thyroid metabolism, and antioxidant activities.

Use in Parkinson's

Levels of these micronutrients are often reduced in aging. These micronutrients are reported to be decreased, unchanged, or increased in people with PD.

Shampoos containing selenium and zinc (e.g., dandruff shampoo) can help oily flaky skin or seborrhea of the scalp and forehead, which is a common complaint.

Precautions

Supplemental zinc can deplete copper, so look for a 10-to-1 ratio of zinc to copper if you take a multivitamin. Copper deficiency results in blood cell problems and, rarely, peripheral neuropathy.

Guidance

There is no evidence to support zinc or selenium supplementation for PD.

Vitamins B1, B6, B12, and Folate

Description and Mechanism of Action

These are the major B vitamins important to cell health, immunity, and energy production.

Vitamin B1 or thiamin is involved in the production and use of glucose for energy. It is important for muscle, brain, and heart health. Deficiencies are rare but can be seen with malnutrition and excessive alcohol use.

Vitamin B6 or pyridoxine is involved in fat metabolism, red blood cell health, immune health, and production of niacin (another vitamin). Of particular

---

[1] The DASH diet is a low salt, high potassium and magnesium diet helpful for high blood pressure and heart disease. Learn more at dashdiet.org.

importance is the role that vitamin B6 plays in the production of amino acids and neurotransmitters such as gamma-amino butyric acid (GABA), serotonin, norepinephrine, and even dopamine.

Vitamin B9 or folate is needed to produce new cells. Low folate levels during pregnancy can increase birth defects related to impaired fetal nerve cell development in utero.

Vitamin B12 is needed to produce new cells, including blood cells.

Use in Parkinson's

The B vitamins are important players in the maintenance of healthy brain cells. Reduced levels of B vitamins have been linked to various brain conditions such as seizures, stroke, migraine, pain, dementia, Alzheimer's, and PD.

The B vitamins are important to PD health. People with diets highest in B6 have lower risk of PD. This protective effect is stronger in smokers than non-smokers. Low vitamin B12 is linked to cognitive difficulties, and folate deficiency is linked to depression.

Among the additional neurologic problems:

- Vitamin B12 deficiency can be associated with cognitive decline, anemia, fatigue, and neuropathy and balance problems. The elderly, people with pernicious anemia, those using certain gastric reflux medicines or antacids, and strict vegetarians are at greater risk for deficiency.
- Folate and B6 deficiency can be associated with depression and poor response to antidepressant therapy.

A deficiency in vitamin B6, folate, or B12 can increase levels of the amino acid homocysteine. Homocysteine is also produced in the metabolism of levodopa and can be elevated by the category of medicines used to treat PD called catechol-o-methyl-transferase (COMT) inhibitors (e.g., entacapone, Comtan®, Stalevo®, tolcapone, Tasmar®). Elevated levels of homocysteine can cause problems such as:

- Blood clotting problems
- Stroke
- Heart disease

The figure illustrates how both folate and vitamin B12 participate in the metabolism, essentially reducing homocysteine levels; conversely, the increase in homocysteine that occurs as the PD medicine levodopa is metabolized.

Precautions

High levels of vitamin B6 can interact with the dopaminergic medicines monoamine oxidase (MAO) inhibitors (rasagiline and selegiline) and block the absorption of levodopa. The National Institutes of Health (NIH) set the upper limit of vitamin B6 for adults to 100 mg daily. Doses higher than 200 mg have been associated with peripheral nerve toxicity with symptoms of numbness and painful or burning feet and hands. Recommended daily dosage is less than 15 mg daily.

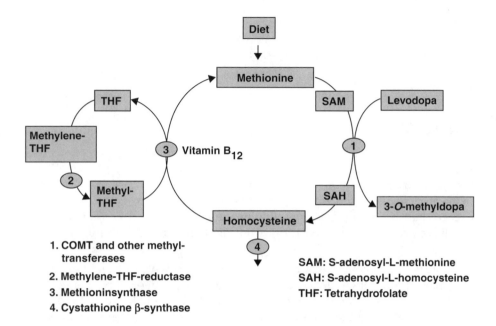

1. COMT and other methyl-transferases
2. Methylene-THF-reductase
3. Methioninsynthase
4. Cystathionine β-synthase

SAM: S-adenosyl-L-methionine
SAH: S-adenosyl-L-homocysteine
THF: Tetrahydrofolate

Vitamin B12 supplements should be avoided in people with Leber's or optic neuropathy. Vitamin B12 can cause a skin rash and unmask certain problems such as polycythemia vera (associated with high red blood cell count) and gout. Ask your cardiologist or primary care doctor about B vitamins if you have heart disease requiring angioplasty and/or arterial stents, as studies suggest that B vitamins can increase re-blockage.

Vegetarians may find it difficult to get vitamin B12 in their diet. Vitamin B12 requires stomach acid for absorption across the stomach wall. Antacids and medicines used for acid reflux or heartburn can reduce B12 absorption. Older patients are at risk for pernicious anemia, a condition in which vitamin B12 absorption is limited, so injections are used instead of oral supplements.

Guidance

B vitamins are included in most multiple vitamin products and sold separately as vitamin B complex. Repeated studies fail to show a benefit of taking vitamin B pills in the absence of deficient levels but do show benefits when vitamin B is elevated through diet. Limit alcohol use, since excessive alcohol use can reduce vitamin B levels. As always, aim to get your vitamins through the food you eat rather than relying on a vitamin pill as the sole source.

Foods rich in B vitamins:

- Vitamin B1 is found in pork, wheat and rye flour, kidney beans, and wheat germ.
- Vitamin B6 is found in cheese, milk, eggs, beans/legumes, potatoes, fish, meat, flour, grains, carrots, and peas.

- Vitamin B9 (folate) is found in fortified cereals and products baked with fortified flour, leafy green vegetables, fruits such as bananas and melons, legumes, yeast, liver, and mushrooms.
- Vitamin B12 is found in dairy products, meat, fish, and shellfish.

ANTIOXIDANTS

As you have learned, dopamine nerve cells are especially vulnerable to oxidative stress (you may wish to review the section on oxidative stress in Chapter 3). Antioxidants occur naturally in the body to protect cells from oxidative damage. However, when antioxidant stores are depleted or oxidative stress levels exceed their buffering capacity, cell damage and disease are possible. Fortunately, you can replenish declining antioxidants through diet to minimize this damage.

There is a lot of controversy about whether supplements truly fight disease in the absence of a known deficiency. The largely unregulated supplement industry is driven more by marketing claims of improved health, longevity, and well-being that far exceed the scientific evidence. This is the case for antioxidants, the sale of which is often based on chemical research in the laboratory and not in the body.

The undisputed fact is that antioxidants are an important part of cellular health. What is disputed is whether a supplement offers the same benefits. Once again the evidence to date favors food over pills. Here are just a few reasons why antioxidants from foods are superior to antioxidants derived from a pill:

- *Dose and Delivery:* Rapid absorption of pills into the bloodstream will lead to abnormally high peaks in concentration rather than the more controlled absorption that happens when ingested as food. Alternatively, some supplements will be poorly absorbed when not ingested with foods, as noted with fat soluble supplements. Also, designing a pill with multiple antioxidants in the ratios ideal for our bodies is difficult if not impossible to achieve. A varied diet can offer this diversity in natural amounts.
- *Chemical Structure:* The chemical structure of vitamins is sometimes similar to but not the same as, or in the same proportion as, that found naturally in foods. Examples include vitamin E and vitamin A. The synthetic forms can have different and/or toxic effects.
- *Synergistic Effects:* Other healthful vitamins or chemical agents found together in food can lead to synergistic effects that are greater than that measured for individual compounds. For example, vitamin E and C when ingested together have greater health benefits through their antioxidant actions than when ingested alone. These natural combinations found in food are hard to approximate in pill form.
- *Other Combined Benefits:* You can assess a product by the company it keeps. Foods highest in vitamins and minerals also tend to have healthier fats, proteins, fiber, and carbohydrates, leading to combined health benefits.

- *Lifestyle Change:* People who choose diets based on their abundance of a particular vitamin or supplement may pay greater attention to their overall health, eat healthier foods in general, and live a healthy lifestyle.

Given the superiority of food over supplements, let's start by learning about antioxidant foods before reviewing more common supplements. The Antioxidant Food Shopping List (provided in Part V, Personalize Your Care) will help you to increase your dietary antioxidants.

Antioxidant Potent Diet
Description and Mechanism of Action
An antioxidant potent diet is one that emphasizes fruits, vegetables, and whole grains. Antioxidants from diet include vitamin E, C, beta-carotene (vitamin A) and polyphenols. Polyphenols are complex molecules found in fruits, vegetables, and whole grains. They are important to the health of plants by regulating hormones and resisting damage from ultraviolet radiation, bacterial invasion, and the harmful results of cellular toxins. Polyphenols impart color to food and work synergistically as antioxidants to buffer the oxidative stress produced as a by-product of cellular metabolism. A diet rich and varied in color is likely to have both a higher and more varied amount of antioxidants (do not be fooled, though, by artificial coloring added to many foods). Compare the colors (and antioxidant potential) of the following two meals:

1. High: Salmon, beats, green salad with tomatoes and peppers, berries
2. Low: French fries, bread, hamburger, ketchup, lettuce, and cookies

Use in Parkinson's
The Mediterranean diet is particularly high in antioxidants. This diet shows many health benefits including lowering risk of heart disease, high blood pressure, cancer, diabetes, PD, dementia, stroke, and depression.

Precautions
Getting your antioxidants in foods ensures you are getting them in their natural state and with other antioxidants that work together synergistically when combined. Antioxidants in pill form are sometimes synthesized in a non-natural state, do not represent the balance found in nature, and can sometimes serve as toxic pro-oxidants when taken alone in high amounts.

Guidance
Nutritional research consistently shows health benefits from *diet* over supplements. Observe the natural colors of food on your plate—but remember that some foods are artificially colored, such as some fish, beverages, cereals, and baked goods. The following tips can increase the antioxidant potential of your diet:

- Eat the colors of the rainbow to ensure a variety of antioxidants. Usually the stronger the color the greater the potential.

- Use olive oil (extra virgin when flavor allows) over regular oils and fats.
- Choose dark green leafy vegetables such as spinach and arugula instead of iceberg lettuce for your salad.
- Increase your daily servings of fruits, vegetables, and whole grains.
- Choose high-quality chocolate (more than 70% cocoa) over milk chocolate.
- Drink green tea (decaffeinated is available, if needed).
- Add flaxseed to food.
- Choose grass-fed beef and meat.
- Substitute colorful beans (e.g., pinto, black beans) for meat as a source of protein.
- Choose fruit over baked goods for dessert.
- Eat fresh, frozen, and local foods when possible. Antioxidant levels decline if produce is not picked ripe and the longer food sits on the grocery shelf, delivery truck, or your refrigerator.
- Take advantage of farmer's markets to improve the freshness and variety of foods and control the pesticides you eat.

The Antioxidant Food Shopping List in the last chapter of this book will help you to make the best dietary choices.

Glutathione and N-Acetyl Cysteine
Description and Mechanism of Action
Glutathione is a tripeptide (three amino acids: glutamate, glycine, and cysteine) produced by the body. Glutathione is a powerful antioxidant that could potentially protect against cellular damage produced by oxidative stress. Both oxidative stress and mitochondrial dysfunction are linked to cellular damage in PD.

N-acetyl cysteine is a precursor to glutathione. N-acetyl cysteine increases the production of glutathione in the body and supports mitochondrial energy metabolism in animal studies. Magnetic resonance spectroscopy shows increased glutathione levels in the brain of people with PD after receiving a single dose of N-acetyl cysteine, showing that this supplement is converted to glutathione in the brain.

Use in Parkinson's
Glutathione is a potent antioxidant in the brain. It is reduced with age and in many chronic conditions including PD. Since glutathione is composed of three amino acids (building blocks of protein), it cannot be taken in pill form since it is metabolized in the gastrointestinal tract in the same way that proteins are broken down. Intravenous and intranasal forms do exist to aid absorption into the bloodstream and brain.

Interest in glutathione for PD continues since it is a powerful antioxidant that is reduced in the substantia nigra of people with PD long before symptoms are significant. Intravenous glutathione improved motor symptoms in a small four-week placebo-controlled study. Results were modest and returned to baseline at the end of the study.

N-acetyl cysteine is an option in pill form since it is converted to glutathione in the body.

Precautions

Glutathione in pill form is a popular supplement sold over the counter as a health supplement to support many brain conditions including PD. This is an example of the marketing influence and power behind the multibillion-dollar supplement industry, since glutathione in pill form is not absorbed by the body and therefore is not effective.

Intravenous glutathione produced by compounding pharmacies is available at various specialty centers. This therapy carries risk associated with injection, is not covered by health insurance, and is very expensive. Only one small placebo-controlled study has been done to support use of this therapy, and the results were modest. In general, intravenous therapies have a higher risk than their oral counterparts. There is one scientific report of a case study of severe liver damage noted in a Japanese man while taking glutathione that reversed after stopping this supplement. Because of all this evidence, this therapy is not recommended.

Novel methods of administration such as intranasal use may prove helpful. Researchers are currently investigating whether this method of use is safe and effective for PD symptoms.

Guidance

Oral glutathione is not effective. Risk and cost of intravenous administration appears to outweigh the benefit. Current studies evaluating safer methods of administration such as intranasal spray are underway. Dose and benefit of N-acetyl cysteine is also not clear and studies are underway to test this supplement in PD. In summary, limited evidence is available to support the use of these compounds at present, but hopefully future studies will offer more definitive guidance.

Inosine
Description and Mechanism of Action

Uric acid is a chemical compound formed by the breakdown of purines in the body. Purines are major components of all cells and form the building blocks of the gene molecules, DNA and RNA. Purines are chemicals found in many foods, especially protein. Inosine is a uric acid precursor that is used to increase levels of this compound.

Uric acid and inosine are powerful antioxidants and anti-inflammatory agents. Inosine also binds to brain adenosine receptors thought to be an important neuromodulator in PD. Findings of altered uric acid levels in people with PD have encouraged scientists to explore these chemicals as potential treatments for PD.

Use in Parkinson's
Uric acid is reduced in people with PD and interestingly this correlates with disease duration. Slower decline in motor symptoms is associated with increased uric acid levels. What's more, higher uric acid levels are associated with lower need for levodopa and higher brain dopamine as determined by DaTSCAN imaging.

Studies confirm that inosine, as a powerful antioxidant and anti-inflammatory agent, can increase blood and spinal fluid levels of uric acid, which further supports recent studies evaluating this compound as a treatment for PD.

Precautions
High uric acid levels can cause gout, a painful form of arthritis. High levels can also cause kidney stones. Risk of kidney stones increases with dehydration and can cause severe pain and kidney damage.

Guidance
Further studies are needed to understand the relationship between uric acid and PD. These studies will be an important first step in determining whether uric acid is a neuroprotective agent capable of protecting vulnerable nerve cells or is a biomarker that can measure disease state/severity or produce a finding not directly related to disease but instead some other associated change that coexists with PD.

Clinical experts do not recommend inosine at this time, given these uncertainties and the potential risks of elevated uric acid.

Foods high in purines that can increase blood urate levels:

- Anchovies
- Dried beans and peas
- Meat, especially organ meats
- Alcohol

Vitamins A, E, and C
Description and Mechanism of Action
Vitamins A and E are fat soluble and vitamin C is a water soluble vitamin. These vitamins have strong antioxidant properties. Preformed vitamin A is different from beta-carotene, a natural vitamin A precursor found in foods.

Use in Parkinson's

Diets high in vitamin E and carotenoids are associated with lower risk of PD. Analysis of multiple studies suggest that diets high in vitamin E but not vitamin C or carotenoids can protect against PD. These varied results are common in studies aiming to correlate vitamin use or ingestion and disease risk. The complexity of vitamin studies and treatment is highlighted in findings that vitamins in combination have different effects than vitamins in isolation, further supporting the quality benefit of foods over pills. For instance, certain ratios of vitamin C, E, lycopene (found in tomatoes), and carotenoids when combined produced higher antioxidant activity than when consumed in isolation.

Precautions

A diet rich in a specific vitamin is very different from taking the vitamin(s) isolated in a pill. This idea, sometimes called food synergy, describes the additive health benefits when nutrients are consumed in combination. A focus on diet may take more effort but is certainly more effective and safer.

Vitamins A and E (as well as vitamins D and K) are fat soluble vitamins and high doses can lead to toxic levels in the body. A meta-analysis of multiple studies analyzing the effects of vitamin E suggest that high-dose vitamin E increases mortality. Similarly, high doses of vitamin A can cause headaches, seizures, and osteoporosis; furthermore, high doses carry risk to the fetus if taken in pregnancy. Unlike beta-carotene in foods, preformed vitamin A found in supplements can be toxic a high levels.

Guidance

Adhere to the concept of food synergy—that is, vitamins in combination and in their natural form—offer better antioxidant and health benefits than artificial ratios and chemical derivatives found in many vitamin/supplements. Certain foods are particularly rich in these antioxidants.

Foods rich in vitamin A (carotenoids) include:

- Sweet potatoes
- Carrots
- Green leafy vegetables
- Winter squash

Foods rich in vitamin E include:

- Green leafy vegetables
- Peppers
- Asparagus
- Nuts and seeds, especially almonds, peanuts, and sunflower seeds
- Avocados
- Olives and olive oil

- Tomatoes
- Kiwi
- Apricots

Foods rich in vitamin C include:

- Citrus
- Yellow peppers
- Green leafy vegetables
- Brussels sprouts
- Cauliflower
- Guava
- Strawberries
- Pineapple

INTERVIEW WITH THE EXPERT: NUTRITION AND SUPPLEMENTS

A NUTRITION SCIENTIST TALKS ABOUT FOOD, HEALTH, AND PARKINSON'S

Why is nutrition important to health?

The word nutrition comes from the Latin root, nūtrīre, *to nourish*. All living things must be *nourished*, and the field of nutritional neuroscience is attempting to figure out what nourishes the brain. Nutrients are those things that we obtain from our environment that are essential to human health and function. If there is evidence that human health suffers without it, it's a nutrient. Genes, environment, age, gender, medications, and disease status all contribute to individual nutritional requirements.

While food is a tremendous source of nutrients, nourishment comes from non-dietary sources, too—the organisms in our intestines, sunlight, air, gravity, sleep, and social connections are all examples of nutrients.

Can supplements take the place of a healthy diet or vice versa?

A healthy diet is essential, but a healthy diet alone is not enough. As we fortify salt with iodine to prevent goiter and mental retardation,

(continued)

INTERVIEW WITH THE EXPERT (continued)

there are some circumstances where diet is simply not enough. There are some nutrients we don't obtain through diet, like oxygen and vitamin D.

Whereas healthy adults are able to make enough of their own glutathione and coenzyme Q10, there is evidence that individuals with PD may not be able to produce enough of these nutrients. While it has not been studied, it's unlikely anyone can eat enough asparagus and avocado to meet their glutathione needs or consume enough animal hearts to obtain Q10.

To complicate matters further, some pharmaceutical drugs influence nutritional requirements. For instance, levodopa depletes the body of folic acid, which drives up blood levels of an amino acid called homocysteine. While normal in low doses, elevated homocysteine has been linked to increase incidence of dementia in PD. This doesn't make levodopa a bad drug. It means that if you're on levodopa, you should talk to your provider about adding folate to your diet or whether you need a folic acid supplement or a homocysteine level check.

What are the top foods for Parkinson's?

Green tea, black tea, coffee—three or more cups daily. Smelling it is just as important as drinking it.

Fresh herbs and spices: Ideally, grow your own herb garden. Get in the habit of adding pepper, curry, turmeric, cinnamon, clove, rosemary, and thyme to your meals.

Fish: Small, oily fish—such as mackerel, smelt, herring, and anchovies—are sustainably harvested; eat them, but not fried.

Fruits and vegetables: Go for color and diversity. Try to eat what grows in your area when it's in season. Foods to emphasize include eggplant, tomatoes, strawberries, blueberries, avocados, kale, collards, bok choy, and asparagus.

Nuts, seeds, and beans: Legumes are a great source of fiber and antioxidants, promoting the growth of healthy intestinal flora, which impacts everything from constipation to brain inflammation.

Avoid fried foods, processed foods, unnecessary calories, pesticides, and artificial sweeteners. Beef, pork, milk, and cream should be consumed in moderation.

(continued)

INTERVIEW WITH THE EXPERT (*continued*)

What simple steps can Parkinson's individuals take to enhance their diet?

- Only put things in your mouth that nourish you. Too often, we eat out of habit, boredom, anxiety, depression, or celebration. Don't be afraid to break old habits and try new ones.
- Your plate should be as colorful and fresh as possible.
- Chew food slowly and eat with friends.
- Avoid overeating, especially if you are overweight. Many of the benefits of calorie restriction can be obtained by not eating for three hours before bed.

Laurie K. Mischley, ND, MPH

Dr. Mischley is a naturopathic doctor practicing in Seattle, WA. She recently completed her doctoral training in nutrition sciences from the University of Washington. Her area of expertise surrounds conditionally essential nutrients in PD.

ANTI-INFLAMMATORY AGENTS

Inflammation is caused by infection, immune system reactions, tissue damage, cellular degeneration, and cell damage from toxins. Chronic inflammation is associated with many diseases including arthritis, heart disease, cancer, dementia, multiple sclerosis, neuropathy, and stroke. Inflammation also accompanies nerve cell death in PD, and this inflammation can potentially influence the cascade of changes that are associated with disease progression.

Foods can be pro-inflammatory or anti-inflammatory. For this reason, we begin with a discussion of the anti-inflammatory diet, followed by a discussion of a few supplements noted to have anti-inflammatory effects.

Anti-Inflammatory Diet
Description and Mechanism of Action
An anti-inflammatory diet includes foods that reduce inflammation and excludes foods that cause inflammation. Foods that are particularly pro-inflammatory include saturated fats, transfat, certain oils, and refined and simple sugars. These foods produce inflammatory chemicals called cytokines. Fats can also oxidize and enhance oxidative stress. Excessive glucose can chemically alter cell membranes, a process called glycosylation associated with aging and hormonal balance.

Use in Parkinson's

Many of the principles of an anti-inflammatory diet are also part of the Mediterranean diet, which is associated with a decreased risk of PD and other brain conditions such as dementia, depression, and stroke.

Precautions

Always seek medical advice or guidance before making any significant dietary changes. Getting the variety of foods and nutrients you need when making dietary changes can be difficult, especially if it means different foods, different cooking and preparatory techniques, and different food combinations than you are accustomed to. You may benefit from advice from a nutritionist.

Guidance

A balance and varied diet that is low in processed foods, saturated fats, and refined sugars and high in fruits, vegetables, and non-meat sources of protein is ideal.

Choose these foods:

- Salmon, walnuts, purslane, and flax as sources of omega-3 fats
- Olive oil instead of vegetable oil or prepared salad dressings
- Fruits and vegetables
- Ginger, turmeric, onions, and garlic
- Nuts
- Soy
- Low-fat dairy

Omit or limit these foods:

- Red meat
- Fried foods
- Refined and simple carbohydrates
- Fructose corn syrup
- Gluten and dairy (if you have an allergy to these foods)
- Excessive alcohol

Omega-3 Fatty Acids, Fish and Krill Oil
Description and Mechanism of Action

Omega-3 fatty acids are essential fatty acids, meaning they are necessary for cell health but not synthesized in the body. We must therefore get all of our omega-3 fatty acids from foods. Omega-3 fatty acids are important for general health. These fats are associated with reduced risk of heart disease, diabetes, cancer, arthritis, and reduced blood clotting. These fats also play an important role in the development of nerve cells.

Omega-3 fatty acids make up part of the cell's outer membrane and help keep cells fluid and stable. Omega-3 fatty acids also reduce inflammation by shifting chemical reactions away from omega-6 producing inflammatory prostaglandins and arachidonic acid. There are three important types:

- Alpha-linolenic acid (ALA) found in some vegetables and vegetable oils
- Eicosapentaenoic acid (EPA)
- Docosaheaenoic acid (DHA)

Your body does convert (albeit inefficiently) some ALA into DHA and EPA. Fish and fish oil are the main sources of omega-3s (DHA/EPA) in the diet.

Use in Parkinson's

Diets high in omega-3 are possibly associated with a lower risk of stroke, depression, cognitive decline, and Alzheimer's disease. At present, there is no direct connection between PD and omega-3 fatty acids, but studies remain limited. Fish oil with and without antidepressants improved PD depression in a placebo-controlled study. In addition, omega-3 fatty acids proved to have neuroprotective effects in an animal model of PD and reduced dopamine cell death caused by the neurotoxin 1-methyl-4-phenyl-1,2,3,6-tetrahydropyridine (MPTP).

Precautions

High doses of fish oil can increase bleeding risk. Avoid fish oil if you are allergic to fish. Vegetarian sources of omega-3 are available but may not have the same potency. As always, it is important to choose your supplements carefully. The supplement you select should be pure and devoid of toxins such as mercury (commonly found in fish) and lead.

Guidance

Omega-3 fatty acids are found in cold water, oily fish such as salmon, mackerel, sardines, herring, halibut, and tuna. Other foods include some forms of algae, flaxseed, canola oil, soybeans, pumpkin seeds, and purslane. Walnuts are high in ALA, which can be turned into DHA and EPA by your body.

Make sure you are taking the correct dose if your doctor recommends fish oil. The total amount of fish oil advertised on the front of the package is different from the amount of omega-3 (DHA and EPA) contained in the supplement. Typical doses range from 1,000 to 1,500 mg daily combined DHA/EPA. Be sure to check the amount of DHA and EPA by reading the label.

Krill oil is obtained from small sea-living crustaceans. Krill is reported to have higher concentrations of EPA and also contain the potent antioxidant astaxanthin.

Be sure to keep fish oil and all oils out of the heat and sun to avoid oxidation and toxic by-products. You may wish to keep these products in the refrigerator or freezer (which also reduces unpleasant "fishy burps").

Vegetarians should consider adding ground flaxseed to their diet instead of flax oil. Flaxseed adds healthy fiber and potent antioxidant lignans to your diet.

Probiotics
Description and Mechanism of Action
Probiotics are bacteria or yeast that coexist in our intestinal tract to maintain healthy function. Problems occur when this healthy balance is disrupted by the presence of foreign or disease-causing bacteria. This imbalance can cause changes in gastric motility, increasing symptoms of bloating and constipation, inflammation of intestinal lining, and leakage of unwanted chemicals and toxins into the bloodstream. Researchers are taking this one step further suggesting there is a connection between bacteria, gastrointestinal function, and brain activity. Alteration in gastrointestinal bacterial can affect brain functions such as emotions, cognition, and pain. The influence of gastrointestinal bacteria, inflammation, and altered absorption on brain activity is called leaky gut, leaky brain.

Probiotic supplements are used to restore this balance in favor of healthy bacteria.

Use in Parkinson's
Early pathological changes in PD are found in the nose and gastrointestinal tract, perhaps long before brain changes occur. This finding poses two interesting questions:

- Are environmental toxins—inhaled or ingested—responsible, in part, for PD?
- Are there preventive measures that can limit damaging effects of these toxins at the intestinal level?

Probiotics could serve a role to reduce inflammation and absorption of unwanted chemicals. A study of newly diagnosed PD individuals found that increased levels of gram negative bacteria are associated with increased intestinal alpha-synuclein (cellular changes associated with PD) and gut leakage. These studies are in their infancy and more research is needed to determine if there is a clear relationship between intestinal bacteria, inflammation, and PD.

Probiotics may also work by reducing PD symptoms. Treatment with lactobacillus reduced symptoms of bloating, abdominal pain, and sensation of incomplete colon emptying in PD individuals suffering from constipation. Probiotics could also improve motor symptoms by reducing small intestine bacterial overgrowth. Small intestine bacterial overgrowth is seen in PD; a recent study suggesting its occurrence in over 25% of individuals studied and contributing to worsening motor scores and increased off time.

Precautions
Side effects from probiotics are minimal, including mild bloating. However, there could be risk of infection when introducing bacteria to your diet, especially if you have an underlying immune condition. It has not been shown that probiotic

supplements truly reset the natural balance of healthy intestinal bacteria and yeast in the same way as foods. Just because a bacteria is deemed "healthy" does not mean that it will have healthful effects if ingested alone and in the high concentration often found in pills.

Guidance

There is no guidance to support use of a particular probiotic product or dose. The aforementioned study used lactobacillus, a bacteria found in dairy products. Studies in healthy women suggest that adding a daily serving of yogurt to the diet can improve measures of emotion and cognition. Until more guidance is available, simply eating yogurt will add healthy protein, calcium, and probiotics to your diet. Other food sources of probiotics include kombucha, kefir, sauerkraut, pickles, and fermented foods.

Turmeric

Description and Mechanism of Action

Curcumin is a polyphenol with strong anti-inflammatory and antioxidant properties that is found in the turmeric root. Turmeric contains about 5% to 10% curcumin. Turmeric is an important ingredient in Indian cooking (responsible for the yellow color of curries) and has been used as a medicinal herb for centuries. Interest in curcumin stems in part from the very low rate of Alzheimer's disease in India and the speculation that this spice may play a role in that finding. Researchers note that turmeric reduces memory decline and beta-amyloid plaque formation, a pathological feature in Alzheimer's disease.

Turmeric is under active study for many conditions given its strong antioxidant and anti-inflammatory properties. Some of the conditions or symptoms being studied are:

- PD
- Alzheimer's and related dementias
- Traumatic brain injury
- Cancer
- Arthritis
- Gastrointestinal conditions such as ulcers, inflammatory bowel disease, and indigestion

Use in Parkinson's

There is no direct evidence that turmeric improves PD-related symptoms or delays or treats related brain pathology. Studies to date show many promising effects, though these studies are performed in animals or isolated nerve cells in the laboratory. Nonetheless, some of the exciting evidence or ways that turmeric could potentially influence pathological changes associated with PD are by:

- Fighting oxidative stress and restoring mitochondrial function and depleted glutathione (a powerful antioxidant)
- Protecting against toxic effects of the misfolded protein alpha-synuclein
- Protecting animals from neurotoxin-induced MPTP parkinsonism
- Exerting pharmacological action similar to medicines such as monoamine oxidase type B (MAO-B) inhibition

Precautions

Turmeric can lower blood sugar, especially when combined with glucose-lowering drugs used to treat diabetes, and increase risk of bleeding. Turmeric can also interact with medicines used to reduce stomach acid such as omeprazole, esomeprazole, and lansoprazole.

Guidance

Turmeric is not easily absorbed through the gastrointestinal tract and the blood-brain barrier. Ingesting turmeric with food, especially fats, can help absorption into the blood and then brain. The enzyme bromelain (an enzyme found in pineapple that can break up proteins) and black pepper increase absorption of turmeric, so many turmeric products contain them as well. How much curcumin is needed to exert anti-inflammatory and antioxidant effects is unknown. Dosages range from 80 mg to 1,500 mg daily. Dosages of 80 mg lipidated curcumin (a proprietary blend designed to improve absorption) had positive effects on multiple health measures when given to healthy adults. There is no dose determined for people with PD.

BIOENERGETICS

Bioenergetics are a group of compounds that serve to improve energy production in the cell. Bioenergetics can influence PD cell health by:

- Increasing nerve cell energy production
- Increasing muscle energy storage

Mitochondria are organelles or structures in the cell that serve to produce energy important for cell life. Energy is produced through a cascade of chemical reactions in a process called electron transport. PD is associated with mitochondrial deficiency at one step in this chain of energy-producing chemical reactions. There are multiple cofactors or chemicals that participate in mitochondrial energy production along this chain. An increased level of these cofactors may, in part, support energy production in the setting of this deficit.

Muscle contraction requires energy, so energy must be stored for everyday use in the muscle. Compounds such as creatine serve to store energy needed for muscle contraction and strength.

Coenzyme Q10
Description and Mechanism of Action
Coenzyme Q10 (CoQ10) is a supplement and chemical found in food and the body. CoQ10 is an antioxidant that may protect nerve cells from damage and is an important factor in mitochondrial energy production. As you know, mitochondria produce cell energy important for biochemical activities and cellular health. Mitochondrial dysfunction and impaired energy production are linked to cellular damage associated with PD. Interest in CoQ10 for PD is based on these important functions and the finding that this molecule decreases with age and PD.

Use in Parkinson's
A small placebo-controlled study suggested that 1,200 mg CoQ10 slowed negative changes in the activity of daily living by 44% over 16 months. Participants also received a 1,200 mg IU daily dose of vitamin E to aid absorption and antioxidant activity. This led to a large NIH-sponsored, multicenter trial evaluating higher doses of CoQ10 and its potential disease-halting effect in people with mild disease not yet requiring dopaminergic medicine for symptom control. Six hundred participants received either placebo, 1,200 mg, or 2,400 mg daily and were evaluated over a 16-month period or until dopaminergic medicine was needed. This much-anticipated study was halted in 2011 when an early analysis showed no difference in motor testing between CoQ10 and placebo treatment and a slight but not significant decline in the CoQ10-treated individuals.

Precautions
CoQ10 is generally well tolerated. Mild side effects include abdominal discomfort, decreased appetite, nausea, and diarrhea. Taking the supplement with food can reduce or eliminate these side effects. CoQ10 could potentially reduce blood glucose levels and affect clotting ability, so it should be used with caution if you are taking a blood thinner or have diabetes. Some researchers believe that statins, a group of medicines used to treat high cholesterol, can reduce levels of CoQ10.

The cost of CoQ10 is high and this is an important "side effect," especially if the cost of a treatment influences purchase of other proven treatment choices such as traditional medicine, rehabilitation, food selection, exercise, or relaxation therapies.

Guidance
Research to date identifies no clear benefits associated with CoQ10 and PD. CoQ10 is actively studied in other conditions such as heart disease, diabetes, cancer, prevention of statin myopathy (muscle damage associated with certain cholesterol medicines), and aging.

As discussed throughout this book, the answer may not lie simply in the use of a supplement like CoQ10, but in the favorable effects noted when combinations of these healthy agents and lifestyle are taken together. Factors such as genetics, age, stress, comorbid medical problems, and other toxic exposures are likely to vary from one person to another and could potentially impact the effect of these supplements. For example, scientists are exploring the role of exercise on oxidative stress and the normal antioxidant response to exercise—since exercise itself is an antioxidant and antioxidant pills may disrupt this natural adaptive balance. Whether these findings can hold true from the laboratory to the person and to diseases such as PD is not certain. What combination and factors are ideal is not known and indeed very difficult to study. The best approach is a practical and scientifically sound defense—optimize the diet as nature has intended and you optimize the defense.

CoQ10 is an example of a supplement that may differ from one product to the next. Because this supplement is fat soluble, absorption can vary based on foods eaten, time of day taken, other supplements taken at the same time, and the type of CoQ10 used. Ubiquinone CoQ10 is converted through a biochemical process in the body to ubiquinol CQ10, a form that is more readily used by the body. Ubiquinol CoQ10 is available as a supplement, although these supplements were not used in the clinical research described. Vitaline® was the brand name used in the aforementioned clinical trial and is ubiquinone CoQ10 packaged in a patented formula with vitamin E to aid absorption.

Coconut Oil and Medium Chain Fatty Acids
Description and Mechanism of Action
Coconut oil is abundant in medium chain fatty acids. These fats are different from long chain fatty acids, which are the more common type of fats in American diets. The difference is in the size of the molecule—specifically, the length of the carbon chain that makes up the chemical backbone of fats. Medium chain fatty acids contain 6 to 12 carbon molecules while long chain fatty acids have over 14 carbon molecules. Another difference is the way the body metabolizes these fats. Medium chain fatty acids are metabolized to ketone bodies. Ketone bodies are an energy source for the brain; in fact, the brain uses ketones preferentially and more efficiently than glucose.

There is significant interest in ketogenic diets and medium chain fatty acids for Alzheimer's disease. The ketogenic diet includes little to no carbohydrates or sugars. Instead, fats and proteins are converted to energy, most importantly in the form of ketones. Axona® is an FDA-approved medical food for Alzheimer's that contains medium chain fatty acids. It increased blood ketone levels and measures of cognitive function in individuals with mild to moderate Alzheimer's disease. Axona® is a medical food and not intended to be a treatment for Alzheimer's.

Hydroxybutyrate is a medium chain fatty acid found to improve cognition in mild Alzheimer's and protect nerve cells in the laboratory from MPTP neurotoxin damage. Hydroxybutyrate is under study for PD.

Use in Parkinson's
Evidence for use of coconut oil and medium chain fatty acids as a treatment for PD or dementia is based solely on individual reports and not backed by clinical studies.

Precautions

Coconut oil may increase triglyceride or cholesterol levels and cause gastric bloating. Some researchers believe coconut oil will increase brain ketone levels only if part of a very strict ketogenic diet and not when added in small amounts to a standard diet.

Guidance

Coconut oil is a flavorful oil that can be added to one's diet. It is solid at room temperature and can add smooth texture to blended drinks and desserts. Coconut oil is fairly stable and also has a high smoking point, so it is a good oil for cooking. Look for virgin rather than refined coconut oil. Refined coconut oil often uses a chemical process to remove scent and fatty acid levels.

Creatine
Description and Mechanism of Action

Creatine is a naturally occurring amino acid found in foods (especially meat) and the body with greatest concentration in muscle. Creatine is converted to phosphocreatine, which in turn participates in cellular energy production. Creatine supplements are used by athletes to boost performance in high-intensity exercises and to increase lean muscle mass. Interest in creatine for PD goes beyond muscle building. Creatine can increase mitochondrial energy production, prevent neurotoxic effects of MPTP in animal models of parkinsonism, and exert antioxidant properties.

Use in Parkinson's

Interest in creatine for use in PD focuses on the two possible benefits:

1. Improved mitochondrial energy production and nerve cell health
2. Improved muscle mass and strength

To date, there is no evidence to support the hypothesis that creatine's antioxidant or energy-enhancing actions are neuroprotective. An analysis of two controlled trials did not show benefit of creatine over placebo on motor symptoms or quality of life in PD. A large NIH-sponsored, multicenter trial studied 1,741 people with PD and the effect of 5 g of creatine taken twice daily. The National Institute of Neurological Disorders and Stroke (NINDS) halted the study in 2013 when an early analysis showed no difference between supplement and placebo.

Creatine can potentially boost the strengthening effects of an upper body weight lifting program in PD individuals, enhancing muscle mass and strength in older individuals. This could prove beneficial for exercise tolerance, fatigue from weakness, and motor performance.

Precautions
There were no safety concerns identified in the large NIH study of over 1,700 people using a specific brand of creatine. However, this may not be true for all brands available over the counter. High doses can decrease blood sugar and cause water retention and kidney disease. Do not use creatine if you have diabetes or kidney disease. There are reports of contaminated creatine and at least one case report of rhabdomyolysis (muscle damage) and kidney failure.

Guidance
Creatine may improve strength and muscle mass. Talk to your health care provider before starting creatine.

NADH
Description and Mechanism of Action
Nicotinamide adenine dinucleotide (NADH) is produced from vitamin B3. NADH assists in the production of energy or adenosine triphosphate (ATP) in cellular mitochondria and in the synthesis of dopamine. You will remember that PD is associated with dysfunction of mitochondria, which impacts cell energy production. Research in NADH for PD is fueled by the idea that energy production will be improved if this and other energy production cofactors (assistance molecules) are increased.

Use in Parkinson's
The theoretical rationale behind use of this supplement is to boost cellular energy and dopamine production. NADH therapy improved motor symptoms and related inability as well as medicine on time (duration of medication dose effect) in open label (non-placebo-controlled) studies. However, placebo-controlled studies have different findings. Intravenous and intramuscular treatment with NADH improved motor symptoms to the same degree as placebo.

Precautions
Placebo-controlled studies do not support claims of benefit in open label studies. NADH is unstable and it is possible that many over-the-counter NADH pills are not effective. There are no significant side effects (other than cost) identified with doses of 5 mg twice daily.

Guidance
There is no evidence to support use of NADH in the absence of deficiency. NADH deficiency is unusual but can be associated with vitamin B3 deficiency in alcoholics.

IMMUNO- AND NEUROMODULATORS

These group of chemicals have complex actions at the cellular level and, unlike classic neurotransmitters, work with other neurochemicals to fine-tune or modulate nerve activity. Immune function, hormonal control, circadian rhythms, and neurotransmitter activity are examples of the complex physiologic processes influenced by these agents.

Melatonin and Tryptophan
Description and Mechanism of Action
Melatonin is a neuro-hormone responsible for regulation of circadian rhythms. Circadian rhythms are physiologic, neurochemical, and behavioral cycles that occur on an approximate 24-hour cycle. Specifically, melatonin regulates the sleep-wake cycle that helps us sleep at night and maintain alertness during the day. Melatonin is made from tryptophan through a pathway that includes the amino acid tryptophan, which is converted to 5-hydroxy tryptophan (5HTP) and serotonin then finally to melatonin by enzymes activated at night.

Melatonin is also a powerful antioxidant. Evidence shows that this hormone increases important antioxidants such as glutathione and protects dopamine nerve cells from MPTP-induced neurotoxic damage. Melatonin secretion is reduced in people with PD, especially those with excessive daytime sleepiness. There appears to be a phase shift of nighttime melatonin elevation in PD compared to people without the disease, but it is not clear if it is caused by the disease itself or dopaminergic medicines.

Use in Parkinson's
Melatonin is sometimes used to aid sleep. Modest improvements in PD-associated sleep quality were experienced with 5 mg and 50 mg doses, with 50 mg showing more favorable results. Melatonin 3 mg to 12 mg can also reduce REM sleep disorder.

Precautions
The safety of higher doses (greater than 3 mg) is not established. Early-morning sedation, depression, and vivid dreaming are experienced by some. Melatonin can alter blood sugar levels in diabetes and influence the immune system. Some medicines interact with melatonin, including sedatives, blood pressure medicines, and blood thinners so be sure to talk to your health care provider before using this (or any) supplement.

Guidance
Low dose melatonin (1 mg to 12 mg) can be used for sleep and REM sleep disorder. Melatonin is available in regular and extended release formulations. Extended release formula may be an alternative for the more common problem of early-

morning awakening and fragmented sleep. Other therapies that can alter melatonin include:

- Exercise
- Bright light therapy (see Chapter 9)
- Tryptophan

Vitamin D
Description and Mechanism of Action
Vitamin D is a fat soluble vitamin of particular interest for bone health, given its role in regulating calcium absorption in bone and tissues. Vitamin D plays an even larger role in health with recent findings linking vitamin D levels to blood pressure regulation and reducing risk of cardiac disease, psoriasis, diabetes, and cancer. Vitamin D is also categorized as a neuro-hormone given its importance in regulating key neurologic functions. Research now links deficiency of this vitamin to multiple sclerosis, dementia, and cognitive function, PD, and falls.

Use in Parkinson's
Vitamin D deficiency is linked to PD. Higher levels of vitamin D is associated with a reduced risk of developing PD. People with PD were measured to have lower levels of vitamin D when compared with people with Alzheimer's disease or "healthy" persons. The low levels measured in people with early disease did not change with disease progression, leading to yet more questions about the role of this vitamin in PD-related pathology. A vitamin D receptor gene is being actively studied as a PD susceptibility gene.

Other ways that vitamin D can be important to people with PD health include:

- Decreased risk of bone fracture from falls
- Reduced risk of depression and cognitive decline with aging
- Reduced falls

Precautions
Use vitamin D with caution and only under the supervision of your health care provider especially if you have liver disease, kidney disease, hypoparathyroidism, malabsorption syndrome, sarcoidosis, and possibly other granulomatous diseases, as you may have increased sensitivity to the effects of vitamin D. Vitamin D is a fat soluble vitamin that is stored in fatty tissue. Toxicity from high dose supplementation can occur with all fat soluble vitamins. A blood test is available to monitor changes in vitamin D with treatment. Toxic levels of vitamin D can cause:

- Kidney stones or damage
- Nausea or vomiting
- High blood calcium and sedation

- Weakness and fatigue
- Calcification in blood vessels (atherosclerosis) and other non-skeletal tissue

Guidance

Vitamin D is sometimes called the "sunshine vitamin" because it is produced when skin is exposed to ultraviolet rays in sunlight. Ten minutes of sunshine a day can help increase your levels of vitamin D. Sun exposure does increase risk of skin cancer and the risk of melanoma, a malignant form of skin cancer. This risk is higher in people with PD. Talk to your primary care doctor about the role of a dermatologist (if you do not already have one) on your health care team.

You may have low levels of vitamin D in winter months, if you live in northern states, or if you have intestinal malabsorption syndromes such as cystic fibrosis or celiac disease or have had intestinal surgeries. A simple blood test, 25-hydroxy vitamin D [25(OH)D] test, can determine if you are deficient and help with follow-up treatment. Be aware that the cost of this test is not always covered by medical insurance. The Institute of Medicine has concluded that a 25(OH)D level of 20 ng/mL (50 nmol/liter) or above is adequate for bone health.

There are two important forms of vitamin D:

- D2 (ergocalciferol), which is a synthetic form found in many over-the-counter supplements and prescription forms of vitamin D
- D3 (cholecalciferol), which is the natural form of vitamin D

Both forms must be converted in the body to a usable form of vitamin D, but vitamin D3 is converted more efficiently and therefore is more potent. At least one study suggests that these two forms are not equal in their benefits. Vitamin D3 but not D2 reduced mortality in a meta-analysis of 50 studies, including almost 95,000 people (mostly older women).

Talk to your health care provider about vitamin D and whether a blood test is needed to measure your level.

Vitamin D is present naturally in only a few foods, so it is often added (fortified) to foods.

Foods rich in vitamin D include:

- Cold water fish such as salmon, tuna, sardines
- Cod liver oil
- Eggs
- Vitamin D fortified milk and cereal
- Vitamin D fortified milk substitutes, such as soy, rice, and almond milk

NEUROCHEMICALS AND AMINO ACIDS

Neurochemicals and amino acids are important for cell structure and neurotransmission. For example, some amino acids, which are the building blocks of protein, also play a role in the synthesis of neurotransmitters including dopamine, serotonin, acetylcholine, GABA, and norepinephrine. These neurotransmitters regulate mood, movement, sleep, cognition, relaxation, and alertness, making them very important to brain function and PD.

CDP-Choline (Citicholine)
Description and Mechanism of Action
CDP-choline (citicholine) is a member of a class of compounds called phospholipids. Phospholipids are an important part of cell membranes, including nerve cells. Citicholine is important for growth and repair of cells and exerts antioxidant effects in laboratory studies. Citicholine may be reduced in PD as a result of dopamine decrease and also appears to increase dopamine levels, which of course raises interest in this supplement as a treatment for PD.

Use in Parkinson's
Double-blind studies are small but suggest that citicholine is superior to placebo, resulting in a 23% and 33% improvement in bradykinesia and rigidity, respectively. Citicholine was tested in 85 people with PD treated with their usual dose or half their usual dose of levodopa. There were no significant differences between the two groups even though the citicholine group received only half of their usual levodopa dose. This suggests that this supplement can help reduce levodopa dose and side effects.

Citicholine is more widely used for cognitive symptoms. A review of studies analyzing the effect of citicholine for cognitive symptoms in Alzheimer's, PD, or stroke-related dementia suggests this supplement may improve cognitive function.

Precautions
Citicholine appears to be safe. Side effects are mostly gastrointestinal such as nausea, bloating, and gastric pain.

Guidance
Most studies use doses up to 400 mg three times daily. Studies are brief and only tested a small number of individuals, so evidence for its benefit is limited.

GABA
Description and Mechanism of Action
GABA plays an important role in relaxation and reducing the impact of stress and muscle tone. GABA also plays a key role in the treatment of seizures, anxiety, insomnia, and muscle spasticity. GABA serves to inhibit neural activity between cells as the primary inhibitory neurotransmitter in the brain and spinal cord. GABA is an important neurotransmitter in the basal ganglia with notable actions including the regulation of dopaminergic activity in animal models of PD. High

strength MRI measures increased GABA levels in the putamen region of the basal ganglia in people with mild to moderate PD. Conversely, loss of dopaminergic nerve cells in PD leads to decreased GABA activity in the subthalamic nucleus (STN). The resulting reduced GABA inhibition of this nucleus, in turn, leads to excessive STN nerve cell activity. Deep brain stimulation of the STN region is thought to reduce this excessive activity. This information suggests that GABA plays an important but complex role in the pathology and motor control of PD.

Use in Parkinson's
GABA is an amino acid that serves to modulate important motor circuits. Unfortunately, GABA is not noted to improve motor symptoms, most likely due to the complex changes and varied effects in different areas of the basal ganglia motor circuitry. GABA is often used instead to improve sleep and anxiety. Information on dosing is based on anecdotal reports and not research-specific evidence.

Precautions
GABA is poorly absorbed through the blood brain barrier so entry into the brain is limited. Side effects and drug interactions appear to be minimal.

Guidance
Doses range from 500 mg to 1 g three times daily. Always work with your health care provider to find the right dose for you. Remember that treatment of anxiety and insomnia is an important part of health and well-being with PD, so optimal treatment will likely require a multipronged approach. Do not use supplements alone to treat significant anxiety.

Naltrexone
Description and Mechanism of Action
Naltrexone is an opioid antagonist. Opioid receptors are located throughout the brain and spinal cord and play an important role in regulating pain. Antagonists block the activation of these receptors and are used to treat alcohol and narcotic (opioid) addiction or overdose. Naltrexone at lower dose (4.5 mg) is used in multiple neurologic conditions including PD, multiple sclerosis, and impulse control disorders.

Use in Parkinson's
Naltrexone has been studied as a treatment for movement symptoms of PD, levodopa-induced dyskinesia, and impulsivity control symptoms associated with dopaminergic therapy. Studies tested different doses described in general as low (4.5 mg) and high (greater than 100 mg) dose naltrexone. Most reports of naltrexone's benefit in PD are based on anecdotal or individual experiences that do not

control for diagnosis, symptoms studied, or placebo effect. Overall research suggests that naltrexone (5 mg/kg/day and 100 mg daily) does not improve motor symptoms of PD.

Naltrexone may play a modest role in treatment of dopaminergic complications. High dose naltrexone (250 mg to 350 mg daily) modestly improved levodopa dyskinesia in one small study. Naltrexone in another small study also improved a medicine-induced impulse control problem, pathological gambling, which is otherwise unresponsive to standard therapeutic interventions such as reduction in dopamine agonists or addition of selective serotonin reuptake inhibitors. However, only three individuals were included in this open label case study, and subsequent placebo-controlled studies did not show a benefit.

Precautions
Liver problems have been associated with naltrexone use.

Guidance
There is no support for use of naltrexone, yet this is one supplement that continues to gain a significant following based on individual reports.

Phosphatidylserine
Description and Mechanism of Action
Phosphatidylserine is a member of a class of compounds called phospholipids. Phospholipids are an important part of cell membranes, including nerve cells. Phosphatidylserine plays a key role in cell apoptosis or programmed cell death. Interest in phosphatidylserine focuses largely on cognitive health and dementia. Limited studies have also evaluated this supplement for athletic performance.

Use in Parkinson's
The role of phosphatidylserine in PD is unknown. This supplement did not protect against MPTP neurotoxin-induced parkinsonian cognitive change in animals.

Precautions
Side effects include gastric upset and insomnia at higher doses. Bovine-derived and plant-based supplements are available. Plant-based soy supplements do not carry the risk of bovine-derived supplements (e.g., concern about cow tissue contamination that can cause disease such as mad cow disease).

Guidance
Positive effects of phosphatidylserine are mostly studied with bovine (cow)-derived supplement. Results from soy-based supplements are limited and may have the same results. Doses range from 300 mg to 500 mg daily.

Foods high in phosphatidylserine:

- Soy lecithin
- White beans
- Meat
- Fish

S-Adenosyl-Methionine (SAMe)

Description and Mechanism of Action

This supplement was originally used to treat arthritis pain and later depression when it was observed that mood improved in arthritis sufferers after treatment. SAMe has many functions, including the synthesis and metabolism of neurotransmitters dopamine and serotonin. SAMe is also an integral part of levodopa metabolism and protects cells from toxicity associated with dopamine metabolites. Vitamin B12 and folate deficiency can reduce levels of SAMe.

Use in Parkinson's

The effect of SAMe on depression in PD is mixed. At least one placebo-controlled study did show improvement in mood. This study used a combination of 40 mg pills twice daily and 200 mg daily intramuscular injection. There are no studies examining the effect of SAMe on pain associated with PD.

Precautions

SAMe can worsen anxiety and symptoms of bipolar disease, especially mania. SAMe does interact with some medicines. This caution should not be overlooked because SAMe is most often used for depression or pain and medicines used for these symptoms can interact with this supplement. SAMe could interact with the PD medicine levodopa by increasing its metabolism and reducing the amount that enters the brain. SAMe increases serotonin and should be used with extreme caution with other antidepressants, especially serotonin reuptake inhibitors that increase this neurotransmitter. This supplement should be used with caution if you are taking the PD medicines selegiline (Deprenyl®, Zelapar®) or rasagiline (Azilect®) or certain pain medicines such as meperidine (Demerol®) and tramadol (Ultram®), since the combination can cause serotonin syndrome[2].

Guidance

Doses for depression and arthritic pain range from 400 mg to 800 mg divided into three daily doses. SAMe is expensive. Expense, coupled with potential medication interactions, may limit its usefulness.

---

[2] Serotonin syndrome is a potentially serious condition characterized by fever, mental confusion, heart arrhythmia, and muscle excitability seen as twitching and shaking.

Tryptophan and 5-Hydroxy Tryptophan (5HTP)
Description and Mechanism of Action
Tryptophan is an amino acid involved in the synthesis of serotonin and melatonin. Melatonin is an important neuro-hormone for regulation of sleep and circadian rhythm. Serotonin regulates sleep, mood, and anxiety. Tryptophan's synthesis of serotonin is illustrated in the following:

$$\text{Tryptophan} \longrightarrow \text{5-Hydroxy tryptophan (5HTP)} \longrightarrow \text{Serotonin} \longrightarrow \text{5-Acetyl 5HTP} \longrightarrow \text{Melatonin}$$

An analysis of 108 studies evaluating the use of tryptophan on mood or sleep revealed only two with sufficient quality to judge effects. Tryptophan did improve mood compared with placebo, suggesting a small but true benefit. Similar analysis showed conflicting results when measuring impact on mood, sleep, and cognition, further suggesting that results vary based on individual deficiencies in serotonin state or levels.

Use in Parkinson's
Tryptophan depletion is a technique used to reduce serotonin brain levels. A study comparing PD individuals to people without the condition showed a mild change in mood after tryptophan depletion in both groups, but no difference between groups, suggesting that PD depression is not associated with a unique serotonin deficiency. Overall data are inconclusive as to use of tryptophan to treat PD-associated sleep problems or depression.

Precautions
Tryptophan side effects do exist. Tryptophan and 5HTP are metabolized to serotonin in the liver, potentially causing symptoms of anxiety, jitteriness, and heart valve disease. Similarly, tryptophan should be used with caution along with medicines such as antidepressants designed to boost serotonin levels. Eosinophilia-myalgia syndrome was associated with tryptophan use in the late 1980s. Investigation proved it was associated with impurities in the product manufactured by a specific company and not tryptophan itself. This is an important reminder that supplements can carry additional safety risk based on impurities and unsafe manufacturing processes.

Guidance
Tryptophan is usually available in 500 mg and 1000 mg strengths and is taken in divided doses two to three times daily. However, dose for effect has not been established. Tryptophan can be increased by diet rather than supplement. Combining foods high in tryptophan with a small amount of carbohydrate such as crackers or fruit may be a simple aid for difficulty falling asleep. Carbohydrates increase absorption of tryptophan across the blood-brain barrier, allowing more

tryptophan to enter the brain. Findings of increased motor and cognitive reaction time after tryptophan treatment may be a concern for people with PD. This slowing of response time was thought to be related to the sedating effect of this supplement.

Foods high in tryptophan:

- Milk and cheese
- Poultry
- Nuts, such as peanuts, and seeds, such as sesame and pumpkin
- Soy and tofu

Tyrosine

Description and Mechanism of Action

Tyrosine is an amino acid that plays an important role in the production of neurotransmitters including epinephrine, norepinephrine, and dopamine. Low levels are associated with low blood pressure, low body temperature, and hypothyroidism. Interest in tyrosine for PD stems in large part from its role in synthesis of dopamine as illustrated in the following:

$$\text{Tyrosine} \longrightarrow \text{Levodopa} \longrightarrow \text{Dopamine}$$

Tyrosine is converted to levodopa via the enzyme tyrosine hydroxylase, and this rate-limiting enzyme is reduced as dopaminergic nerve cells degenerate in PD. Studies are evaluating treatments that change tyrosine hydroxylase activities so that tyrosine can more efficiently be converted to dopamine in PD.

Use in Parkinson's

An early study measured increased dopamine levels in cerebrospinal fluid after 100 mg/kg tyrosine was given to nine individuals with PD. The idea is that increased levels in the cerebrospinal fluid means greater dopamine levels in the basal ganglia and improved motor symptoms. To date, there are no adequate studies that support this hypothesis.

Tyrosine has also been studied to treat orthostatic hypotension (decrease in blood pressure with standing that is associated with symptoms of dizziness or fainting). Tyrosine given 500 mg twice daily did not help PD-associated orthostatic hypotension.

Precautions

Because tyrosine may interfere with the absorption of levodopa, it should not be taken at the same time as this medicine.

Guidance

It's rare to be deficient in tyrosine. Tyrosine is generally well tolerated.

Foods high in tyrosine include:

- Poultry and fish
- Dairy
- Soy
- Almonds
- Bananas
- Avocados
- Seeds, such as sesame and pumpkin

BOTANICALS

Botanical supplements include plant-based products and herbs used for their healing effect. In this section we will review the more commonly used supplements or plants: marijuana, mucuna pruriens, and St. John's wort. Other commonly used botanical supplements are listed along with their use and potential mechanism of action in the table included within this section.

Marijuana
Description and Mechanism of Action
Marijuana refers to the dried leaves, flowers, stems, and seeds from the hemp plant *Cannabis sativa.* It contains the chemical tetrahydrocannabinol (THC). THC is only one of over 70 cannabinoid compounds found in the plant, each with different biological effects. Collectively, these compounds are similar to natural-occurring chemicals such as anandamide that exist in our bodies and make up the endocannabinoid system involved in brain development and function.

These cannabinoid receptors are located throughout the brain, especially in regions that influence cognition, pleasure, motor coordination, and time and sensory perceptions. High concentrations of cannabinoid receptors exist in the hippocampus (memory), cerebellum (learning and motor coordination), and basal ganglia (motor control). Activation of these receptors results in the "high" that users experience, as well as changes in coordination, problem solving, mood, and altered perceptions such as paranoia or hallucinations.

Marijuana is self-reported to help people manage symptoms of nausea, loss of appetite, muscle spasm and spasticity, pain, and anxiety. There are over 70 identified cannabinoid chemicals in marijuana. These chemical isolates of the marijuana plant have different chemical properties and hence their individual use can be of potential benefit for targeted symptoms. Marinol® is an example of a chemical isolate of marijuana used for a specific medicinal purpose. Marinol® (dronabinol) is synthetic delta-9-tetrahydrocannabinol (delta-9-THC) and an FDA-approved medicine for nausea. Sativex® is a mouth spray approved in Europe for muscle spasticity related to multiple sclerosis (MS) and contains delta-9-THC and cannabidiol (CBD).

Both THC and CBD are powerful antioxidants exerting neuroprotective effects in research models of head injury and neurodegenerative disease. CBD holds promise for medical use since it does not have the psychoactive effects described with the marijuana plant or THC compound. CBD has anti-inflammatory, antioxidant, and immunosuppressive properties measured in the laboratory— properties that may be especially important to brain disease such as MS, head injury, Alzheimer's disease, and PD.

Use in Parkinson's

An early study of five patients with PD showed no change in tremor despite drowsiness, euphoria, and personal accounts of prior beneficial effects. More recently, marijuana use was associated with improved sleep, pain, tremor, and bradykinesia (motor slowness) within 30 minutes after smoking marijuana in clinic.

It is not clear whether the benefits measured in these studies are from a direct effect of marijuana on PD brain chemistry or physiology. Marijuana has a complex neurochemistry with combined psychoactive, behavioral, and motor effects that, alone or combined, can impact tremor and movement. For example, tremor will increase with stress and improve with treatments known to enhance relaxation. Marijuana's behavioral effects may lead to enhanced relaxation and euphoric mood or mitigate the stress response, which alone could reduce tremor.

Precautions

The use of marijuana will likely increase as more states legalize marijuana (at present 23 states permit the medical use of marijuana and 7 states are pending legislative decisions) and as societal attitudes about this drug evolve. Like any drug, marijuana use is not without risk. There are potential negative effects of marijuana and its chemical isolates that should be considered before using.

Behavioral side effects:

- Sedation, apathy, and depression are potential side effects. Apathy and sedation will affect activities such as exercise.

- Psychosis and cognitive changes could be particularly problematic for older people or PD patients prone to hallucinations (also caused by dopamine medicines).

- Change in eating habits are another side effect.

General health effects:

- *Heart:* Heart rate is increased by 20 percent to 100 percent for up to three hours after smoking marijuana, with an increased risk of heart attack one hour after use.

- *Pregnancy:* Marijuana can alter the developing endocannabinoid system in the brain of the fetus. Consequences for the child may include problems with attention, memory, and problem solving.

- *Smoking:* The long-term impact of smoke inhalation and chemical particulates on lung function is unknown.

- *Stroke:* THC causes brain artery constriction and atherosclerosis, which may lead to stroke. Whether this is true for all users is unknown.

Other effects:

- *Overdose and Toxicity:* Medical marijuana is legal in some states but is still an unregulated drug with associated risks including potency, contamination, and impurities. Synthetic marijuana is often laced with other psychoactive compounds to increase the user's high.

- *Addiction and Long-Term Use:* About 9 percent of users become addicted to marijuana. Younger individuals and daily users have an increased risk. Withdrawal symptoms include irritability, sleeplessness, decreased appetite, anxiety, and drug craving.

   Long-term marijuana use can impact memory, learning, judgment and increase the risk of mental illness such as psychosis, depression, and addiction. Impaired judgment and motor coordination can double the risk of a motor vehicle accident, and this risk increases substantially if marijuana is combined with alcohol.

Guidance

The American Academy of Neurology does not sanction the use of marijuana for tremor or other motor symptoms of PD, given the lack of clinical evidence supporting its benefits. Studies are either small, open label without placebo, or based on anecdotal evidence and individual cases. Stress certainly worsens tremor and motor symptoms, and marijuana may indeed have a short-term positive impact on stress physiology. There are, however, other alternatives that are proven to combat stress with fewer side effects. Therapies such as meditation, guided imagery, exercise, and yoga should be considered as treatments with lower risk, especially given their broader general health gains. Marijuana should not be used as a substitute for these holistic approaches to stress management.

As with any drug, there are pros and cons to using marijuana, and it is important to review them with your health care provider. In particular, the potential addictive, psychoactive, and behavioral consequences of marijuana use must be taken into consideration. Nevertheless, specific cannabinoids found in marijuana hold promise as therapeutic agents for neurologic conditions, offering yet another strategy for treatment, especially when traditional medications fail or cause intolerable side effects. The following are important questions to review before considering marijuana:

- Are there other treatments with fewer side effects that can be tried?
- How will side effects such as sedation, depression, or apathy affect my life?
- Do I have cognitive problems, or am I at risk of hallucinations or psychosis?
- Can I abide by restrictions such as not driving under the influence of marijuana?
- Are there occupational considerations or concerns about use around children?

Mucuna Pruriens
Description and Mechanism of Action
Mucuna pruriens or cowhage seeds have been used in India and Ayurvedic medicine for the treatment of PD for thousands of years. The benefits are due to the fact that these seeds contain 3% to 4% levodopa. As such, mucuna pruriens is often referred to as natural dopamine.

Use in Parkinson's
A small controlled study to compare the effect of carbidopa/levodopa and 30 g-dose mucuna pruriens in eight patients with motor fluctuations and dyskinesia showed faster and longer on time without dyskinesia after mucuna treatment. The study's authors propose that benefits from mucuna pruriens may be due to more than just levodopa, given that this treatment did not increase dyskinesia in the same way that carbidopa/levodopa did.

Precautions
Levodopa in mucuna pruriens is chemically similar to that found in carbidopa/ levodopa pills, which means mucuna will also have similar dopaminergic side effects and risks. The levodopa concentration in one bean depends on certain factors such as age, maturity of the seed when harvested, soil composition with harvest, and time in storage. In other words, the amount of levodopa in mucuna (cowhage seeds) differs between seed batches. Also, supplements are not FDA-regulated, so dose, purity, and safety cannot be guaranteed. Therefore, it remains difficult to standardize levodopa dosage from mucuna.

Guidance
Mucuna pruriens contains levodopa and therefore carries the same potential risks and side effects of carbidopa/levodopa (Sinemet®). Since drug levels are variable with mucuna, the benefits and side effect risk from this supplement can be erratic. Talk to your health care provider about the potential risks and benefits of pharmaceutical levodopa before using mucuna pruriens.

St. John's Wort
Description and Mechanism of Action
St. John's wort (*Hypericum perforatum*) is a flowering plant used for its antiviral, anti-inflammatory, and antidepressant properties. Antidepressant effects of St. John's wort are likely due to increased brain levels of serotonin. There is conflicting evidence to support the use of St. John's wort for depression, but this uncertainty was also noted when studying a class of medicines with similar actions, selective serotonin reuptake inhibitors (SSRIs). St. John's wort is generally recommended for mild to moderate depression.

Use in Parkinson's
St. John's wort has not been adequately studied for PD-associated depression.

Precautions
Major depression can significantly impact quality of life, so treatment should be under clinical supervision and not self-directed. Although clinical trials suggest St. John's wort is as safe as or safer than standard antidepressants, it is important to note that these studies are performed with high-grade supplements. Over-the-counter products may not have the same degree of purity and potency, so similar safety claims cannot be made. St. John's wort can interact with many medicines, including other antidepressants, blood thinners, and some pain medicines. This supplement should not be used with the Parkinson's medicines selegiline or rivastigmine (monoamine oxidase type B [MAO-B] inhibitors) due to the increased risk of serotonin syndrome with this combination. Symptoms of potentially life-threatening serotonin syndrome include:

- *Behaviors:* confusion, agitation, irritability, restlessness
- *Autonomic Symptoms:* fever, sweating, elevated heart rate and blood pressure, cardiac arrhythmias, diarrhea
- *Muscle Activity:* twitching, spasm, and tremor

Guidance
Depression can worsen well-being, quality of life, and cognitive and motor symptoms of PD. Optimize your treatment by involving your health care team. Talk with your health care provider or doctor about the best treatments for your mood. Focus on a holistic approach that includes counseling, exercise, dietary changes, and stress reduction.

OTHER COMMONLY USED BOTANICAL PRODUCTS		
NAME	USE	POSSIBLE MECHANISM OF ACTION
Chamomile (German, Roman)	Sleep, anxiety, irritable bowel	GABA
Cinnamon	Decrease food-associated blood glucose levels in diabetes; protective effect in parkinsonian mice	Antioxidant, protein modulation
Cranberry	Prevent bladder infection	Block binding of bacteria to the bladder wall

(continued)

| OTHER COMMONLY USED BOTANICAL PRODUCTS (*continued*) |||
NAME	USE	POSSIBLE MECHANISM OF ACTION
Ginger	Nausea, gastric bloating, and motility	Acetylcholine, serotonin
Ginkgo	Memory	Acetylcholine
Ginseng	Immune health, memory	Dopamine serotonin, acetylcholine, GABA
Kava	Anxiety, insomnia	GABA
Lemon Balm	Anxiety, insomnia	GABA
Licorice	Orthostatic hypotension, acid reflux	Acts on the kidney, increasing sodium retention and blood volume; protects the mucosal lining in the GI tract from inflammation
Peppermint	Indigestion, irritable bowel syndrome	Reduces smooth muscle spasm in the GI tract
Valerian Root	Anxiety, insomnia	GABA

Note: GABA, dopamine, acetylcholine, and serotonin are neurotransmitters.

References
Vitamins and Minerals
Calcium

Bolland, M. J., et al. 2012. "Effect of calcium supplements on risk of myocardial infarction and cardiovascular events: Meta-analysis." *British Medical Journal* 341: 3691.

Iron and Manganese

Guilarte, T. R. 2010. "Manganese and Parkinson's disease: A critical review and new findings." *Environmental Health Perspectives* 118: 1071–80.

Pichler, I., et al. 2013. "Serum iron levels and the risk of Parkinson's disease: A mendelian randomization study." *PLoS Medicine* 10(6): e1001462.

Selenium and Zinc

Zhao, H. W., et al. 2013. "Assessing plasma levels of selenium, copper, iron, and zinc in patients of Parkinson's disease." *PLoS One* 8(12): e83060.

Antioxidants
Glutathione and N-Acetyl Cysteine

Hauser, R. A., et al. 2009. "Randomized, double-blind, pilot evaluation of intravenous glutathione in Parkinson's disease." *Movement Disorders* 24: 979–84.

Holmay, M. J., et al. 2013. "N-Acetylcysteine boosts brain and blood glutathione in Gaucher and Parkinson diseases." *Clinical Neuropharmacology* 36: 103–6.

Naito, Y., et al. 2013. "Glutathione." *Reactions Weekly* 1309: 22.

Inosine

Moccia, M., et al. 2015. "Uric acid relates to dopamine transporter availability in Parkinson's disease." *Acta Neurologica Scandinavica* 131: 127–31.

Sun, C. C., et al. 2012. "Association of serum uric acid levels with the progression of Parkinson's disease in Chinese patients." *Chinese Medical Journal* 125: 583–87.

Vitamins A, E, and C

Chen, J., et al. 2009. "The scavenging capacity of combinations of lycopene, beta-carotene, vitamin E, and vitamin C on the free radical 2.2-diphenyl-1-picrylhdrazyl (DPPH)." *Journal of Food Chemistry.* 2009 33: 232–45.

Etminan, M., et al. 2005. "Intake of vitamin E, vitamin C, and carotenoids and the risk of Parkinson's disease: A meta-analysis." *Lancet Neurology* 4: 362–65.

Miller, E. R., et al. 2005. "Meta-analysis: High dose vitamin E supplementation may increase all-cause mortality." *Annals of Internal Medicine* 142: 37–46.

Miyake, Y., et al. 2011. "Dietary intake of antioxidant vitamins and risk of Parkinson's disease: A case control study in Japan." *European Journal of Neurology* 18: 106–13.

Anti-Inflammatories
Omega-3 Fatty Acids, Fish, and Krill Oil

Bousquet, M., et al. 2007. "Beneficial effects of dietary omega-3-polyunsaturated fatty acid on toxin-induced neuronal degeneration in an animal model of Parkinson's disease." *Journal of the Federation of American Societies for Experimental Biology* 22: 1213–25.

———. 2011. "Impact of omega-3 fatty acids in Parkinson's disease." *Aging Research Reviews* 10: 453–63.

Moralex, T., 2008. "Depression in Parkinson's disease: A double-blind, randomized, placebo-controlled study of omega-3 fatty-acid supplementation." *Journal of Affective Disorders* 111: 315–19.

Probiotics

Cassani, E., et al. 2011. "Use of probiotics for the treatment of constipation in Parkinson's disease patients." *Minerva Gastroenterologica e Dietologica* 57: 117–21.

Cryan, J. F., and T. G. Dinan. 2012. "Mind-altering microorganisms: The impact of the gut microbiota on brain and behavior." *Nature Reviews Neuroscience* 13: 701–12.

Fasano, A., et al. 2013. "The role of small intestinal bacterial overgrowth in Parkinson's disease." *Movement Disorders* 28: 1241–49.

Forsyth, C. B., et al. 2011. "Increased intestinal permeability correlates with sigmoid mucosa alpha-synuclein staining and endotoxin exposure markers in early Parkinson's disease." *PLoS One* 6: e28032. doi:10.1371/journal.pone.0028032

Tan, A. H., et al. 2014. "Small intestinal bacterial overgrowth in Parkinson's disease." *Parkinsonism and Related Disorders* 20: 535–40.

Tillisch, K. 2013. "Consumption of fermented mild product with probiotic modulates brain activity." *Gastroenterology* 144: 1394–410.

Turmeric

Balusamy, J. 2008. "Curcumin treatment alleviates the effect of glutathione depletion in vitro and in vivo: Therapeutic implications for Parkinson's disease explained via in silico studies." *Free Radical Biology and Medicine* 44: 907–91.

DiSilvestro, R. A., et al. 2012. "Diverse effects of a low supplement lipidated curcumin in healthy middle-aged people." *Nutrition Journal* 11: 79.

Mishra, S., and K. Palanivelu. 2011. "The effect of curcumin (turmeric) on Alzheimer's disease: An overview." *Pharmacological Research* 63: 439–44.

Rajeswari, A., and M. Sabesan. 2008. "Inhibition of monoamine oxidase-B by the polyphenolic compound curcumin and its metabolite tetrahydrocurcumin in a model of Parkinson's disease induced by MPTP neurodegeneration in mice." *Inflammopharmacology* 16: 96–99.

Zhaohui, L., et al. 2011. "Curcumin protects against A53T alpha-synuclein-induced toxicity in a PC12 inducible cell model for Parkinsonism." *Pharmacological Research* 63: 439–44.

Bioenergetics
Coenzyme Q10

Gomez-Cabrera, M. C. 2008. "Moderate exercise is an antioxidant: Upregulation of antioxidant genes by training." *Free Radical Biology and Medicine* 44: 126–31.

Parkinson Study Group QE3 Investigators. 2014. "A randomized clinical trial of high-dosage coenzyme Q10 in early Parkinson disease. No evidence of benefit." *JAMA Neurology* 71: 543–52.

Shults, C. W., et al. 2002. "Effects of coenzyme Q10 in early Parkinson disease: evidence of slowing of the functional decline." *Archives of Neurology* 59: 1541–50.

Coconut Oil and Medium Chain Fatty Acids

Henderson, S. T. 2009. "Study of the ketogenic agent AC-1202 in mild to moderate Alzheimer's disease: A randomized, double-blind, placebo-controlled, multicenter trial." *Nutrition and Metabolism* 6: 31.

Kashiwaya, Y. 2000. "D-β-Hydroxybutyrate protects neurons in models of Alzheimer's and Parkinson's disease." *Proceedings of the National Academy of Science* 97: 5440–44.

Reger, M. A., 2004. "Effects of B-hydroxybutyrate on cognition in memory-impaired adults." *Neurobiology of Aging* 25: 311–14.

Creatine

Devries, M. C., and S. M. Phillips. 2014. "Creatine supplementation during resistance training in older adults: A meta-analysis." *Medicine and Science in Sports and Exercise* 46: 1194–203.

Hass, C. J., et al. 2007. "Resistance training with creatine monohydrate improves upper-body strength in patients with Parkinson disease: A randomized trial." *Neurorehabilitation and Neural Repair* 21: 107–15.

Xiao, Y., et al. 2014. "Creatine for Parkinson's disease." *Cochrane Database of Systematic Reviews* 17: 6.

NADH

Birkmayer, W., et al. 1989. "The coenzyme nicotinamide adenine dinucleotide (NADH) improves the disability of parkinsonian patients." *Journal of Neural Transmission* 1: 297–302.

Dixdar, N., et al. 1994. "Treatment of Parkinson's with NADH." *Acta Neurologica Scandinavica* 90: 345–47.

Swerdlow, R. H. 1998. "Is NADH effective in the treatment of Parkinson's disease?" *Drugs and Aging* 13: 263–68.

Immuno- and Neuromodulators

Melatonin and Tryptophan

Antolin, I., et al. 2002. "Protective effect of melatonin in a chronic experimental model of Parkinson's disease." *Brain Research* 943: 163–73.

Aurora, R. N., et al. 2010. "Best practice guide for the treatment of REM sleep behavior disorder (RBD)." *Journal of Clinical Sleep Medicine* 6: 85–95.

Dowling, G. A. 2005. "Melatonin for sleep disturbances in Parkinson's disease." *Sleep Medicine* 6: 459–66.

Fertl, E. 1991. "Circadian secretion pattern of melatonin in Parkinson's disease." *Journal of Neural Transmission: Parkinson's Disease and Dementia Section* 3: 41–47.

Mayo, J. C., et al. 2005. "Melatonin and Parkinson's." *Endocrine* 27: 169–78.

Srinivasan, V. 2011. "Therapeutic potential of melatonin and its analogs in Parkinson's disease: Focus on sleep and neuroprotection." *Therapeutic Advances in Neurological Disorders* 4: 297–317.

Videnovic, A., et al. 2014. "Circadian melatonin rhythm and excessive daytime sleepiness in Parkinson's disease." *JAMA Neurology* 71: 463–69.

Vitamin D

Bischoff-Ferrari, H. A. 2009. "Fall prevention with supplemental and active forms of vitamin D: A meta-analysis of randomized controlled trials." *BMJ* 339: b3692.

Bjelakovic, G. 2014. "Vitamin D supplementation for prevention of mortality in adults." *Cochrane Database Systematic Reviews* 1: CD007470. doi:10.1002/14651858 .CD007470.pub3

Butler, M. W., et al. 2011. "Vitamin D receptor gene as a candidate gene for Parkinson disease." *Annals of Human Genetics* 75: 201–10.

Evatt, M. L., et al. 2008. "Prevalence of vitamin D insufficiency in patients with Parkinson disease and Alzheimer disease." *JAMA Neurology* 65: 1348–52.

———. 2011. "High Prevalence of hypovitaminosis D status in patients with early Parkinson disease." *Archives of Neurology* 68: 314–19.

Knekt, P., et al. 2010. "Serum vitamin D and the risk of Parkinson disease." *Archives of Neurology* 67: 808–11.

Tang, B. M. P., et al. 2007. "Use of calcium or calcium in combination with vitamin D supplementation to prevent fractures and bone loss in people aged 50 years and older: A meta-analysis." *The Lancet* 370: 657–66.

Wilkins, C. H., et al. 2006. "Vitamin D deficiency is associated with low mood and worse cognitive performance in older adults." *American Journal of Geriatric Psychiatry* 14: 1032–40.

Neurochemicals and Amino Acids

CDP-Choline (Citicholine)

Agnoli, A., et al. 1982. "New strategies in the management of Parkinson's disease: A biological approach using a phospholipid precursor (CDP-choline)." *Neuropsychobiology* 8: 289–96.

Eberhardt, R., et al. 1992. "Citicholine in the treatment of Parkinson's." *Clinical Therapeutics* 12: 489–95.

Milani, M. 2013. "Citicholine as a co-adjuvant treatment in chronic degenerative central nervous system disease and in ischemic stroke: A review of available data." *Online Journal of Medicine and Medical Science Research* 2: 13–18.

GABA

Emir, U., et al. 2012. "Elevated pontine and putamenal GABA levels in mild-moderate Parkinson's detected by 7 Tesla MRS." *PLoS One* 7: e30918. doi:10.1371/journal .pone.0030918

McIntyre, C. C., et al. 2004. "Uncovering the mechanism(s) of action of deep brain stimulation: Activation, inhibition, or both." *Clinical Neurophysiology* 115: 1239–48.

Naltrexone

Bosco, D., et al. 2012. "Opioid antagonist naltrexone for the treatment of pathological gambling in Parkinson disease." *Clinical Neuropharmacology* 35: 118–20.

Manson, A. J. 2001. "High dose naltrexone for dyskinesia induced by levodopa." *Journal of Neurology, Neurosurgery, and Psychiatry* 70: 554–55.

Nutt, J., et al. 1978. "Effect of an opiate antagonist on movement disorders." *Archives of Neurology* 35: 810–81.

Papay, K., et al. 2014. "Naltrexone for impulse control disorders in Parkinson's disease: A placebo-controlled study." *Neurology* 83: 1–8.

Rascol, O., et al. 1994. "Naltrexone, an opiate antagonist fails to modify motor symptoms in patients with Parkinson's disease." *Movement Disorders* 9: 437–40.

Phosphatidylserine

Cenacchi, T., et al. 1993. "Cognitive decline in the elderly: A double-blind placebo-controlled multicenter study on efficacy of phosphatidylserine administration." *Aging Clinical and Experimental Research* 5: 123–33.

Perry, J. C., et al. 2004. "Behavioral and neurochemical effects of phosphatidylserine in MPTP lesion of the substantia nigra in rats." *European Journal of Pharmacology* 484: 225–33.

S-Adenosyl-Methionine (SAMe)

Bressa, G. M., et al. 1994. "S-adenosylmethionine (SAMe) as antidepressant: Meta-analysis of clinical studies." *Acta Neurologica Scandinavica* 154 (supplement): 7–14.

Carrieri, P., et al. 1990. "SAMe S-adenosylmethionine treatment of depression in patients with Parkinson's disease: A double-blind, crossover study versus placebo." *Current Therapeutic Research* 48: 154–60.

Di Padova, C., et al. 1987. "S-adenosylmethionine in the treatment of osteoarthritis." *American Journal of Medicine* 83: 60–65.

Werner, P. 2001. "COMT-dependent protection of dopaminergic neurons by methionine, dimethionine, and S-adenylmethionine." *Brain Research* 893: 278–81.

Tryptophan and 5-Hydroxy Tryptophan (5HT)

Mace, J. L. 2010. "The effects of acute tryptophan depletion on mood in patients with Parkinson's disease and the healthy elderly." *Journal of Psychopharmacology* 24: 615–19.

Shaw, K. A., et al. 2002. "Tryptophan and 5-hydtoxytrypotphan in depression." *Cochrane Database of Systematic Reviews* 1: CD003198. doi:10.1002/14651858.CD003198

Silber, B. Y., and J. A. J. Schmitt. 2010. "Effects of tryptophan loading on human cognition, mood, and sleep." *Neuroscience and Behavioral Reviews* 34: 387–407.

Tyrosine

DiGrancisco-Donoghue, J. 2014. "Effects of tyrosine on Parkinson's disease: A randomized, double-blind, placebo-controlled trial." *Movement Disorders Clinical Practice* 1: 348–53.

Growdon, J. H., et al. 1982. "Effects of oral L-tyrosine administration on CSF tyrosine and homovanillic acid levels in patients with Parkinson's disease." *Life Science* 30: 827–32.

Botanicals

Marijuana

Frankel, J. P. 1990. "Marijuana for parkinsonian tremor." *Journal of Neurology and Neurosurgery* 53: 436.

Koppel, B. S., et al. 2014. "Systematic review: Efficacy and safety of medical marijuana in selected neurologic disorders: Report of the Guideline Development Subcommittee of the American Academy of Neurology." *Neurology* 82: 1556–63.

Lotan, I., et al. 2014. "Cannabis (medical marijuana) treatment for motor and non-motor symptoms of Parkinson's disease: an open label observational study." *Clinical Neuropharmacology* 37: 41–44.

Mucuna Pruriens

Katzenschlager, R., et al. 2004. "Mucuna pruriens in Parkinson's disease: A double-blind clinical and pharmacological study." *Journal of Neurology, Neurosurgery, and Psychiatry* 75: 1672–77.

St. John's Wort

Hypericum Depression Trial Study Group. 2002. "Effect of *Hypericum perforatum* (St. John's wort) in major depression: A randomized controlled trial." *Journal of the American Medical Association* 287: 1807–14.

Linde, K., et al. 2008. "St. John's wort." *Cochrane Database of Systematic Reviews* 8: CD000448. doi:10.1002/14651858.CD000448.pub3

Schrader, E., et al. 2000. "Equivalence of St. John's wort extract (Ze 117) and fluoxetine: A randomized, controlled study in mild moderate depression." *International Clinical Pharmacology* 15: 61–68.

Other Commonly Used Botanical Products

Attele, A. 1999. "Ginseng pharmacology." *Biochemical Pharmacology* 58: 1685–93.

Clouatre, D. L., 2004. "Kava kava: Examining new reports of toxicity." *Toxicology Letters* 150: 85–96.

Jepson, R. G., et al. 2012. "Cranberries for preventing urinary infections." *Cochrane Database of Systematic Reviews* 10: CD001321. doi:10.1002/14651858.CD001321 .pub5

Khasnavis, S. 2014. "Cinnamon treatment upregulates neuroprotective proteins parkin and DJ-1 and protects dopaminergic neurons in a mouse model of Parkinson's disease." *Journal of Neuroimmune Pharmacology* 9: 569–81.

Pertz, H. H., et al. 2011. "Effects of ginger constituents on the gastrointestinal tract: Role of cholinergic M3 and serotonergic 5-HT3 and 5-HT4 receptors." *Planta Medica* 77: 973–78.

Sarris, J., et al. 2011. "Herbal medicine for depression, anxiety, and insomnia: A review of psychopharmacology and clinical evidence." *European Neuropsychopharmacology* 21: 841–60.

CHAPTER

7

Body Therapy

Body therapies focus on body movement, musculoskeletal alignment, massage, or tissue manipulation. Body therapy (including therapeutic exercise) can play an important role in Parkinson's symptom relief. There are many forms and types of body therapies and finding the right one for you can be difficult with so many choices. The ones included in this book represent therapies that have a body of evidence in support of their use in Parkinson's disease (PD), are frequently used by people with PD, or are most frequently discussed by patients in my clinic.

There are a few general principles that apply when considering any body therapy. First and foremost is your safety. Be sure to research your therapist or practitioner. Begin with a review of their credentials, training, and experience. The following suggestions or questions can be helpful:

- Always include your health care provider in your decision to start a body therapy. In addition, a physical therapist can be very helpful in guiding your treatment by suggesting a therapeutic focus, goal, and guidelines for better outcomes and reduced harm.

- What training or certification do they have? Is training informal or are there formal certifications and clinical licenses that must be obtained to practice?

- Does training include knowledge of anatomy, body mechanics, and PD?

- Are there modifications that can be applied for special situations such as arthritis, osteoporosis, back pain, dystonia balance problems, or deep brain stimulation (DBS)?

Of course it is also important to choose therapies that you are interested in or enjoy, and that are targeted to your symptoms. For instance:

- Do you do better in a group setting or individual setting?
- Are you interested in attending a class or finding a therapy you can do at home?
- Does the therapy help non-motor symptoms that you may have, such as pain or depression?
- Is there a low-impact version ideal for joint problems, pain, and arthritis?

Finally, the application to life in balance promoted throughout this book also applies to choice of body therapies. Balance includes the following:

- Are you coupling high-intensity physical activities with therapies that focus on intentional movement, mind-body connection, or motor relaxation?
- Does your therapeutic program include only passive physical activity (i.e., massage or chiropractic, in which therapy is performed "on" you)? If so, how can the result be enhanced by therapies that also focus on active physical movement?
- Does your body work include integration of the senses, emotions, and cognitive challenge?

Some of the therapies detailed in this section were reviewed in Chapter 5 on Lifestyle Medicine. Examples include massage, therapeutic yoga, tai chi, and the Feldenkrais Method®. Many of the therapies covered here are also mind-body therapies or sensory therapies and could just as accurately be included in those sections.

CHIROPRACTIC MANIPULATION
Description and Mechanism of Action
Chiropractic physicians treat disease using the premise that body structure and alignment impact function and therefore symptoms, disease, and health. The spine, spinal cord, and spinal nerves are the primary focus of treatment. Spinal adjustments are the physical manipulation of muscle, ligaments, and tendons to improve alignment. Chiropractic therapy often combines these techniques with other approaches such as electrical stimulation of muscle, massage, relaxation techniques, and nutritional counseling.

Use in Parkinson's
The American Academy of Neurology states that there is no evidence to support manual therapies such as chiropractic manipulation for treatment of PD motor

symptoms. Nonetheless, it is a popular therapy among PD and non-PD patients alike especially for back pain. A comprehensive review of research studies shows that chiropractic care can help pain in the short term, yet no studies either support or refute the use of chiropractic care for long-term pain control. The use of chiropractic manipulation in Parkinson's is limited to case reports and related observational studies. A case study describing a person being treated for back pain in which the chiropractor suspected and referred the patient for neurologic evaluation highlights a very important point: back pain can coexist with PD motor and postural changes. Treatment is often directed at back pain and in this case PD was an underlying cause. As you have learned, the cause of pain in PD is often multifactorial, including dystonia, musculoskeletal joint changes exacerbated by disease or arthritis, achiness from rigidity, and pain related to inactivity. Given the pain syndromes associated with PD, it is likely that many will seek therapy from a chiropractor. Treatment of pain, however, should also be multifactorial and include medical treatment of motor symptoms and physical therapy.

Precautions

There is much controversy in the medical community about the benefits of this therapy and similar controversy exists when examining risks. A prospective study found that 56% of people reported problems within the first three treatments and 13% of patients defined their problem as severe in intensity, yet the study's authors noted no serious problems. Although not common, there are, however, serious risks associated with chiropractic care. Some of these risks are:

- Overuse of x-ray and radiation exposure.
- The expense of repeated treatments.
- Vertebral dissection after cervical manipulation. The vertebral artery travels through the transverse processes in the neck, a bony portion of the vertebral column, on route to the brainstem. Mechanical damage leads to serious and often life-threatening stroke. High-velocity thrusting motions may be more likely to cause this problem.
- Pinched nerve or vertebral disc herniation after manipulation.
- Damage to DBS wires or battery after upper chest, neck, or head treatment.
- Delayed diagnosis of pain when treatment of back pain is thought to be related to musculoskeletal disease. Other causes of bone pain include infection, neurologic disease, and metastatic cancer.

Guidance

Chiropractic physicians must complete a four-year advanced degree, hold the designation of Doctor of Chiropractic (DC), and be licensed to practice within the state in which they work. Insurance sometimes covers this form of treatment, but many insurers do not. Be sure to talk with your medical doctor about chiropractic therapy, the risks and the benefits. Avoid aggressive and high-velocity manipulation especially on your neck. Ask your chiropractor about out-of-pocket costs, your goals for therapy, and the expected number of treatments necessary to feel results.

Remember that the best therapy for pain, especially back pain, is a multifaceted one. Guided exercise with a focus on muscle strengthening, stretching and postural alignment, weight loss, and physical therapy are an important part of the treatment plan for musculoskeletal disease.

CRANIOSACRAL THERAPY

Description and Mechanism of Action

Craniosacral therapy (CST) was developed by osteopathic physician Dr. John Upledger in the 1970s. This therapy uses very light touch over the skull (cranium), face, spine, and pelvis (sacrum) to examine and treat. The idea is that the cranial sutures (thought to fuse early in life) are dynamic and moving. Arterial pulse and pressure and the flow of cerebrospinal fluid causes subtle rhythmic movement in cranial bones. Manipulation is done to regulate this primary respiratory mechanism by changing the dynamic flow of fluid and movement along the bony axis, leading to healing. CST has been targeted as medical quackery given the lack of scientific evidence to support its underlying mechanism of action.

Use in Parkinson's

Many individuals site improvement in their motor symptoms for brief periods of time after CST. There is, however, no evidence in support of this therapy or its use in PD.

Precautions

There is no evidence to support this therapy. Repeated visits are often required, adding cost that is not reimbursed by insurance.

Guidance

I have heard many stories of success from patients who seek this therapy for stress, rigidity, or tremor. Although there is no explanation for effects based on the proposed physiologic explanation for CST, there are explanations for benefit. The power of the therapeutic relationship between practitioner and patient, coupled with gentle healing touch and gentle breathing, will lead to physiologic changes such as an increase in parasympathetic nervous system activity. This in turn will unleash the health benefits of the relaxation response. Also, as we have learned through exploration of the placebo effect, the power of patient and practitioner beliefs can further enhance the emotional and physical well-being that comes with these changes.

Understanding the complex interaction between therapy, practitioner, expectations, and outcome is an important first step in deciding if this therapy (or another therapy) is right for you.

FELDENKRAIS METHOD® AND ALEXANDER TECHNIQUE®

Description and Mechanism of Action

The Feldenkrais Method, named after the engineer and physicist Moshe Felden-krais (1904–1984), is a method of movement that integrates body and mind in an effort to improve coordination, agility, balance, and performance through move-ment. Many movements are learned habits and these habits can be changed to encourage movement patterns with improved efficiency, flow, and ease of move-ment. This awareness and focus can identify maladaptive motor habits, and help in relearning normal movement patterns.

According to the Feldenkrais Institute, the method is different from exercise with its focus on exertion; rather, the approach focuses on movement with ease, minimal effort, and awareness of the whole self through the practice. Maladaptive movement can become effective and these changes are noted at the neurologic level. At a basic level, the Feldenkrais Method improves posture, coordination, flexibility, and suppleness. Moreover, the Feldenkrais Method alleviates pain by minimizing physiological and psychological stress associated with restricted func-tions. Our experiences, illnesses, history, and culture cause changes and adaptive patterns of movement and psychological behavior. Patterns of inefficiency, compromised self-expression, and forgotten ways of feeling can all be improved. Treatment usually begins with antigravity movements done on the floor.

The Alexander Technique® is named after Frederick Alexander, an Austrian-born (1859) singer and performer who experienced voice problems interfering with his performance. Through self-exploration he became aware of certain head and neck positions and posture and movement habits that impacted his voice and expression. Voice, he noted, could be modified through realignment of the body. Treatment usually begins while sitting in a chair or at a table, often in front of a mirror, with a focus on position and posture and controlled movements.

The Alexander Technique and Feldenkrais Method have many similarities and some subtle differences. The Alexander Technique uses a structured hands-on approach for awareness of alignment and body position, while the latter focuses on practitioner guidance and spontaneous and self-generated expression of movement and ease.

Use in Parkinson's

The Feldenkrais Method and Alexander Technique work with coordination, balance, posture, flexibility, and agility of movement. Significant claims for the Feldenkrais Method are not scientifically proven.

Five-week, three times per week Feldenkrais Method–treatment helped mobi-lity and balance compared with a waitlist control group. A study of 93 PD indi-viduals receiving 24 sessions of the Alexander Technique showed improvement in measures of disability, depression, and attitudes toward self-care compared to a group getting massage or no treatment. Remarkably, this effect remained six months after study completion. The focus of the Alexander Technique on upper body postures and voice suggests that it may be of help for speech problems associated with PD. No studies to date have tested this hypothesis. Speech and lung function, however, are coupled, and pulmonary (lung) function can be improved as noted in healthy volunteers primarily through improvement in posture and inhibition of "slumping." No studies specifically tested the effect of the Alexander Technique on gait.

Taken together, the Feldenkrais Method and Alexander Technique may be helpful for posture, breath support, speech, and motor expression.

Precautions

Be sure that your instructor is a certified practitioner. Practitioners of both the Feldenkrais Method and Alexander Technique must undergo extensive training over three to four years. Study includes anatomy but is mostly "hands on" training. However, no clinical prerequisite or education in body mechanics, psychology, or physical therapy is required. Certified instructors can be found through the following resources:

- The American Society for the Alexander Technique, www.amsatonline.org
- The Feldenkrais Institute, www.feldenkraisinstitute.org and www.Feldenkrais.com

Guidance

Both individual and group classes are available. Ten to 30 or more classes may be needed for results. Talk to the practitioners before you begin to be sure that their style works for you.

MASSAGE

Description and Mechanism of Action

Massage is familiar to most of us as a technique used to improve muscle pain and stiffness by rubbing, pressing, and kneading muscles. The history of massage dates as far back as 2700 BC, as one of the oldest forms of medical therapy. The ancient Greeks, Egyptians, and Chinese used this form of therapy to heal. Modern-day massage has returned to its healing roots as it has come full circle emerging from the sports arena to the medical spa, rehabilitation clinic, and finally medical settings such as hospitals and outpatient clinics.

There are many different types of massage and massage techniques. Some focus on relaxation and stress reduction while others focus on muscle and deep tissue relaxation/release. Examples include:

- *Sports and Muscular Tension.* Swedish massage is a common form of massage that applies long, flowing strokes to aid muscle and body relaxation.

Deep tissue massage uses strong pressure to relieve tension in deep tissues. Both of these techniques are commonly used in athletics.

- *Rehabilitation.* Myofascial release is thought to relieve tension in the connective coating around muscle called the muscle fascia. Gentle pressure, trigger-point compression, and stretching are applied to the muscle to release restricted fascia. This treatment is used by many practitioners including physical therapists to reduce muscle spasm, pain, and spasticity that accompanies disease or injury.

- *Medical Massage.* These therapists undergo additional training in the application of massage to medical conditions. Additional treatment goals include pain relief and emotional and stress relief. Board certification and licensure is required.

- *Lymphatic Massage.* Lymph fluid moves from tissue to the blood vascular system through gentle massage of the lymphatic system by muscle contraction. Lymphatic massage uses light, gentle, circular motions (most often in the limbs) to encourage lymphatic flow and swelling. This technique can reduce fluid accumulation and swelling caused by trauma and surgery.

- *Acupressure and Reflexology.* These techniques are covered in Chapter 9 on Energy and Sensory Medicine.

Some forms of massage use heat, aromatherapy, and music to enhance the relaxation effect, further improving the synergistic effect of the mind-body connection. Eastern medicine has introduced techniques such as acupressure. Healing massage uses gentle touch to promote relaxation, an ancient practice that applies focal pressure to specific points in the body similar to acupuncture.

Use in Parkinson's

The benefits of massage therapy are many. Massage does more than ease the pain or tightness of muscles. It is a healing art that promotes relaxation and stress reduction, so important to one's general sense of well-being. Some find it helpful as a supplemental treatment for depression, anxiety, and insomnia. Direct pressure and massage can improve tissue and joint movement, which can increase range of motion and reduce shoulder and back pain often associated with PD.

Clinical studies investigating the benefits of massage in PD show improvement in self-reported daily activities when 30-minute massages are received twice weekly over five weeks, and in well-being, related daily activities, and self-confidence after eight hourly sessions.

Precautions

Even something as simple as massage has risks. The following are just some of the risks:

- *Dystonia.* Deep tissue or aggressive massage should be avoided in people with dystonia since very aggressive massage and muscle stretching can worsen dystonia and related pain. Very gentle massage techniques such as healing massage should be used on muscle areas with dystonia.

- *Positioning.* Avoid body positions that cause pain. For instance, work with your therapists to find a comfortable position if you have pain when you lie on your abdomen or turn your head to one side.

- *DBS.* People with DBS should avoid massage of the scalp, head, neck, and upper anterior chest, as DBS wires and batteries are fragile and can fracture with applied pressure.

- *Lightheadedness.* Low blood pressure can cause dizziness, falls, and even loss of consciousness. You can reduce the effects of lightheadedness by getting up slowly after massage, drinking plenty of water, and sitting down for a few minutes before getting up to leave.

- *Blood Clots.* Massage should not be performed over an area with a recent blood clot (most commonly the arm and leg) to avoid propagation of the blood clot to other areas. Be sure to seek guidance from your health care provider before getting a massage if you have this problem.

- *Cellulitis, Skin Infection, and Ulcers.* Massage of skin that is infected or ulcerated can lead to further tissue breakdown and damage.

Guidance

It is not entirely clear how massage therapy works or how it helps PD. However, there is strong research evidence in support of massage to increase activity in the parasympathetic nervous system to enhance the relaxation response and improve lymph flow and blood circulation.

A medical massage therapist has training in the application of massage to medical conditions and symptoms. Look for a therapist with training accredited by the Commission of Massage Therapy (www.comta.org). The National Certification Board for Therapeutic Massage and Bodywork sets standards for qualifying exams leading to individual board certification as a massage therapist. Most states also require state certification or licensure, ensuring appropriate training and conduct. Ask if your massage therapist has experience with PD, dystonia, other neurologic conditions, or arthritis. Although this does not ensure a therapist's competence, it at least identifies those therapists in tune with the needs of individuals with chronic illness and physical disabilities.

You may also wish to check with your medical insurance provider, as many insurance programs are now including massage therapy in their list of benefits.

MUSIC THERAPY
Description and Mechanism of Action

Music therapy uses song and components of sound such as beat, melody, and tone to promote healing. Music therapy capitalizes on the powerful effect of music on emotions, behavior, energy, and movement. A music therapist is specially trained to use music and sound in clinical settings to promote movement and healing.

Music can activate widespread neuronal brain circuits and stimulate neurotransmitter release such as dopamine.

Use in Parkinson's

Music therapy can help movement in obvious ways. Bradykinesia in particular was improved in a study using music therapy for PD movement symptoms. Walking, freezing of gait, and control of sequential or repetitive movement are improved when coupled with music of a particular beat or cadence. Slow rhythmic movement can also help soothe anxiety, tremor, and dyskinesia. Music therapy can be used to help these PD symptoms:

- Speech problems
- Apathy and motivation
- Energy
- Mood (anxiety and depression)
- Movement
  - Walking, balance, freezing of gait
  - Slowness of movement and flexibility

Precautions

Be sure you work with a music therapist who is certified by the Certification Board of Music Therapy Association (www.cbmt.org). Some states require music therapist to be licensed. Most insurance carriers do not cover music therapy. Ask your music therapist for the cost of sessions before starting and how these treatments will enhance outcomes you could otherwise get from traditional therapies alone that are covered by your medical insurance such as physical therapy.

Guidance

Music therapy can be especially helpful if you have trouble with initiating movement (freezing of gait), poor motivation, or energy. This therapy is different from physical therapy and should be used in concert with, but not instead of, physical therapy. Both focus on movement, but physical therapy will focus on specific musculoskeletal and neurologic problems. Music therapy uses sound-based therapy to help movement, communication, and emotional and social health. Music therapy can be particularly helpful to engage and motivate when depression and apathy are a problem because it enhances cognitive and social engagement for people with cognitive problems. Music therapists can work with physical therapists to improve freezing of gait, which responds to metronome and similar auditory stimulation.

CLINICAL PEARL: EXPLORE THE HEALING POWER OF MUSIC WITH THESE TIPS

- Listen (and move) to different styles of music. Does one *feel* better than the other, entice you to move in a different way, or make it easier to for you to move?
- Categorize songs according to how they make you feel, and copy them to a CD or your phone so that you can play them when needed. For example, music with a marching beat will help you walk. You can also include music selections that make you:
    - Move to a faster beat (to improve your speed of movement)
    - Happy (to help you when you are down)
    - Energetic (to help you when you are fatigued or lack motivation)
    - Sing along (songs with familiar lyrics let you exercise your voice)
    - Feel calm (to help you relax, fall asleep, and reduce tension)
    - Recall the past and good times (music with a history or from a past era can invoke fond memories and cognitive engagement)
- Choose a song or group of songs to play that will motivate and get you ready for a task such as exercise.
- Join (or start) a singing group or chorus such as Tremble Clefs (www.trembleclefs.com), a national program for people with PD and their partners. Participants come together to support one another, perform, and strengthen voice through singing.

TAI CHI AND QIGONG
Description and Mechanism of Action

Tai chi is both an ancient form of martial art and an exercise. Characterized by gentle, flowing movement and meditation coupled with breathing, this form of exercise is becoming increasing popular due to its low impact on joints. Qigong combines breathing with subtle and flowing movement, along with focused attention of the mind to release life energy (chi) and reach a calm state of mind.

Use in Parkinson's

Tai chi is particularly effective due to the combination of balance work: graceful, sweeping, broad, and controlled movements can counter and improve imbalance and the tight and small amplitude movements associated with PD. The slow, flowing movements put minimal stress on joints, making this form of exercise ideal for people with pain and arthritis.

In one study, 159 people with PD participated in a 24-week, twice weekly 60-minute program of tai chi or in stretching or resistance weight training. The tai chi group had overall better balance measures; what's more, these improvements persisted for three months after completion of the study. The changes that occur in body alignment such as ankle sway and postural sway experienced with tai chi may be especially helpful for balance.

Precautions

As with all mind-body therapies it is important to work with a teacher that is trained in the adaptation of this ancient art to you and your symptoms. Slow changes in body position and shifts in posture and center of gravity are helpful exercises to improve your balance, but these movements can also lead to falls if you have balance problems. Look for instructors who can adapt their class to your needs, including chair movements if your balance is significantly affected.

Guidance

You may benefit from tai chi if you like group exercises, have balance issues, and are interested in the challenge of learning new ways to move and perceive movement. Tai chi can also be helpful if you suffer from arthritis and joint pain, due to its low physical impact.

YOGA AND THERAPEUTIC YOGA

Description and Mechanism of Action

Yoga is derived from ancient Sanskrit meaning to join, unite, or yoke. Mind, body, spirit are one. Yoga is a spiritual, mental, and physical practice with roots in India dating over 5000 years ago. Yoga has gained a considerable following in the United States over the last few decades with particular emphasis on Hatha yoga. Hatha yoga uses physical postures, movements, and poses to join the mind and body. Yoga unites the mind and body through physical practice to bring awareness to sensations of the body, thoughts, and emotions.

Therapeutic yoga blends traditional yoga, breathwork, meditation, and guided imagery to promote physical health and emotional healing. Therapeutic yoga programs are often designed to promote relaxation, reduce pain, enhance mood, and support healing in the setting of chronic illness. Therapeutic yoga goes beyond the stretching and strengthening poses of traditional yoga to focus on gentle and restorative poses known to support relaxation and reduce stress through relief of physical strain and tension. Props such as pillows, blankets, and bolsters are used to gently support the body through movements that open up joints and relieve tension. The physical release of tension is coupled with mental release from gentle touch and guided imagery.

Use in Parkinson's

Yoga can help PD through its multiple focus on:

- *Physical:* Postures and poses are designed for gentle stretching to achieve relaxation of muscle tightness and spasm. Improved body mechanics and muscle relaxation are several aspects of the practice that make it a good choice for individuals with PD.
- *Emotional:* Relaxation, positive imagery, and healing touch can improve mood and lessen anxiety.
- *Supportive Healing:* Instruction and touch originate from an intention of healing, empathy, community, and self-acceptance. In this environment you are accepted and okay just the way you are. You can learn to feel your symptoms without the judgment that can sometimes accompany these symptoms.

Precautions

Yoga can cause injury when performed inappropriately. Look for an instructor who is familiar with PD or other neurologic conditions and with whom you feel comfortable and safe. Your instructor should be adept in modifying poses to your ability and pain should not be part of the experience. You can find trained instructors through the International Association of Yoga Therapists (www.iayt.org).

Guidance

Although there are no studies evaluating the effect of therapeutic yoga on PD, its gentle approach and focus on relaxation and compassionate healing are all important benefits that can make a difference, especially if you are feeling pain, anxiety, or depression. Traditional yoga can improve mood in people experiencing depression and it is likely that therapeutic yoga, with its focus on emotional well-being and healing, will have similar results. Part of the healthful benefits of yoga is the effect of learning to "listen to your body." Do not push your body through pain or force postures that put excessive stress on your joints and muscles.

INTERVIEW WITH THE EXPERT: THE FELDENKRAIS METHOD®

A DOCTOR'S JOURNEY FROM GENERAL NEUROLOGIST TO FELDENKRAIS PRACTITIONER

"If you know what you are doing, you can do what you want."

That is what Moshe Feldenkrais said. But if you don't know, it can take longer. And so it was with me. I studied yoga for fifteen years, stretched, did weights and physical therapy. All good in their own way. But my arthritis was getting worse. In 2005, a retired psychiatrist friend of mine suggested I try Feldenkrais Functional Integration, after he noticed me limping as I walked out of yoga class. Eventually I started sessions with a local practitioner and felt lighter on my feet each time. So, with beginner's mind (and beginner's luck), while visiting my son in college in Boulder, Colorado, I crashed the National Feldenkrais Conference in 2007, soaked up glorious embodied learning, and met several famous American Feldenkrais trainers. I wanted to go to the conference again the following year, but by then classes were restricted to trained practitioners.

I had been practicing neurology in Moscow, Idaho. I began *Awareness through Movement* classes after work. I read all of Dr. Feldenkrais's books and in 2009 I met serendipity all over again while vacationing in New York City. I was walking across town on West 26th Street and saw, to my surprise, the face of Moshe hanging from a purple banner on a second-story factory building. It was the Feldenkrais Institute of New York. Needless to say, I marched in and took a class. One of the students told me they were starting a training program . . . in ten days! I was a five day/week neurologist in private practice. Destiny had hung a plum before me, but it was up to me to decide whether to pick it. So I filled out the application to become a Feldenkrais practitioner and changed my work schedule to accommodate frequent trips to New York City.

My fellow students were physical therapists, occupational therapists, philosophers, neuroscience grad students, Orthodox Jews, alternative body workers, yogis, dancers, "housewives of New York," musicians, athletes, engineers, and all nerds in our own particular way. I was the only physician. That helped me when it came to the anatomy and neurophysiology training. What I learned there was to take a trek into my body, to study my own movement patterns—not necessarily to

(continued)

INTERVIEW WITH THE EXPERT (continued)

banish them, but to recognize them, because by seeing my own patterns I would learn what my options were. In other words, I learned to recognize my own movements from the inside out. It meant plumbing myself to examine the way I moved and to see how that knowledge could help teach me about the connection between my brain and body, reflecting my own life history with all its accidents and incidents as a *person*.

I began applying Feldenkrais principles to my patients in little ways, long before receiving my diploma in 2013. I had my patients thinking about how to get up from a chair. Where is your center of gravity? Do you look up or forward? Where do you put your feet? Did you tighten your chest? Where are your hip joints? How do you get up from the floor? Can you roll over in bed without hurting your back? How can gravity help you? How does your right shoulder connect with your left hip when you stride? How do you bend to pick up a paper clip? Could you visualize your heels to help climb stairs?

By the time I graduated I was working in a movement disorder clinic and 85% of my patients had PD. A support group leader invited me to give a class, and I chose a short lesson about turning that employs the eyes and differentiation of gaze and the shoulders, followed by reintegration. As if by magic the audience learned to turn farther. But it wasn't magic. It only seemed to be because it was easier.

I began teaching at my house to a small group of people with PD and then a day at the YMCA. The number of lessons to choose from is almost limitless. Moshe brought the world at least 1,500 complete lessons, ranging from the head to the toes and all points in between. All parts of the body are involved in a lesson. Even if it focuses on the chest, the student comes to see how she uses her hips, jaw, shoulders, heels, and spine all in concert with her chest. She sees them in her homunculus, the complete person in her brain. The lessons bring the connection between these parts to mind as I speak to her and ask her to move in awareness through movement class.

With PD you have to keep moving. And Feldenkrais makes it easier because it connects your skeleton to the motor organization of your own brain. It's not physical therapy. It's learning about your own movement patterns. At the end of a class you will feel refreshed, alive, and so much more aware. And you start seeing your tasks of daily life as less of a chore—not because I have taught you how to do them, but

(continued)

INTERVIEW WITH THE EXPERT (continued)

because you have learned how to see your own self in a new way. You learn how to learn in a Feldenkrais class. So if getting out of a chair was difficult, you will have found out how to eliminate the motor patterns that might have worked against you in bringing your derrière off the chair and into uprightness onto your two dinky little feet. You take that first step.

Barbara Morgan, MD
Board-certified Neurologist and Guild-certified
Feldenkrais Practitioner

Dr. Morgan's practice in Boise, Idaho, focuses, in part, on the care of people with PD and related conditions.

References

Chiropractic Manipulation

Burton, R. R. 2008. "Parkinson's disease without tremor masquerading as mechanical back pain: A case report." *Journal of Canadian Chiropractic Association* 52: 185–92.

Rubinstein, S. M., et al. 2007. "The benefits outweigh the risks for patients undergoing chiropractic care for neck pain: A prospective, multicenter, cohort study." *Journal of Manipulative and Physiological Therapeutics* 30: 408–18.

Suchowersky, O., et al. 2006. "Practice parameter: Neuroprotective strategies and alternative therapies for Parkinson's disease (an evidence-based review)." *Neurology* 11: 976–82.

Walker, B. F., et al. 2010. "Combined chiropractic interventions for low-back pain." *Cochrane Database of Systematic Reviews* 4: CD005427. doi:10.1002/14651858.CD005427.pub2

Craniosacral Therapy

Green, C., et al. 1999. "A systematic review of craniosacral therapy: Biological plausibility, assessment reliability, and clinical effectiveness." *Complementary Therapies in Medicine* 7: 201–7.

Feldenkrais Method® and Alexander Technique®

Emerich, K. 2003. "Nontraditional tools helpful in the treatment of certain types of voice disturbances." *Current Opinion in Otolaryngology and Head and Neck Surgery* 1: 149–53.

Jain, S. 2004. "Alexander Technique and Feldenkrais Method: A critical review." *Physical Medicine and Rehabilitation Clinics of North America* 15: 811–25.

Stallibrass, C., et al. 2002. "Randomized controlled trial of the Alexander Technique for idiopathic Parkinson's disease." *Clinical Rehabilitation* 16: 695.

Massage

Fernandez-Reif, M. 2002. "Parkinson's disease symptoms are differentially affected by massage therapy versus progressive moor relaxation: A pilot study." *Journal of Bodywork and Movement Therapies* 6: 177–82.

Yoga

Colgrove, Y. S., et al. 2012. "Effect of yoga on motor function in people with Parkinson's disease: A randomized, controlled pilot study." *Journal Yoga Physical Therapy* 2: 112.

Krucoff, C., et al. 2010. "Teaching yoga to seniors: Essential considerations to enhance safety and reduce risk in a uniquely vulnerable age group." *Journal of Alternative and Complementary Medicine* 16: 899–905.

Roland, K. P. 2014. "Applications of yoga in Parkinson's disease: A systematic literature review." *Journal of Parkinsonism and Restless Legs Syndrome* 4: 1–8.

CHAPTER

8

Mind-Body

Mind-body therapies work on the premise that the mind, body, and spirit do not exist in isolation and that disease and/or symptoms change when these are out of balance. Best treatment effects occur when combined with attention to mind, body, and spirit. Individuals practice mind-body therapies for many reasons:

- Improved emotional well-being
- Enhanced healing
- Improved performance and symptom control
- Enhanced resiliency
- Inner peace, acceptance, and relaxation
- Increased positivity and outlook

Broadly speaking, almost any treatment can be classified as mind-body if you accompany treatment with an intentional focus of your thoughts, attitude, intention, and emotions. Even medications can have mind-body effects if you incorporate this focus. Remember the placebo effect? The effect of treatment is the sum of true medication effect and the placebo effect influenced by your own beliefs and expectations. With this in mind, each of the body therapies reviewed previously (in Chapter 7) can also be classified as mind-body if practiced with these ideas in mind. Other techniques for sensory and experiential healing (discussed in Chapters 9 and 10, respectively) can also be classified as mind-body techniques.

It can also be said that the opposite is true. Mind-body therapies could also be classified simply as body therapies if performed in that way. For instance, yoga is no different from stretching and calisthenics if the focus is on physical postures alone without "checking in" with body sensations, sensory and emotional changes, imagery, and breathwork that accompany the practice.

Mind-body therapies have the potential to be particularly helpful since they can increase treatment results and enhance resiliency needed to live with a chronic illness.

BIOFEEDBACK

Description and Mechanism of Action

Biofeedback originated in the 1960s and is based on learning theories developed by behavioral psychologists that tie measures of body function to symptoms and symptoms control. Biofeedback often uses machines to measure signals produced by the body or automatic body functions such as muscle contraction, blood pressure, pulse, temperature, or weight. The use of brain waves (EEG) is used in neurofeedback. The participant uses techniques such as muscle relaxation, breathing, visualization, or thoughts to change the recordings.

Use in Parkinson's

Biofeedback can be useful to reduce muscle tension, pain, insomnia, stress, or anxiety. Specific problems that may respond to biofeedback that are common in Parkinson's disease (PD) include urinary incontinence and bowel or defecation problems. Speech therapists are now using neurofeedback to improve problems with speech and swallowing.

Precautions

There are few risks associated with biofeedback. Not all states regulate the practice of biofeedback. Of concern are the growing number of individuals offering biofeedback without appropriate training. Like all mind-body therapies, it is important to ensure that you are working with a trained professional. Begin by talking to your health care provider about a referral to a specialist in biofeedback. The Association for Applied Psychophysiology and Biofeedback (www.aapb.org) lists individuals trained to perform this therapy.

Guidance

Biofeedback is often performed by psychologists, physicians, nurses, and physical and occupational therapists. Certification for psychologists and medical professionals is available through the Biofeedback Certification International Alliance (www.bcia.org). Three types of certification are available: biofeedback, neurofeedback, and pelvic muscle dysfunction biofeedback. Bowel and bladder therapy (pelvic muscle dysfunction biofeedback) uses biofeedback to improve the coordinated control of pelvic floor and sphincter muscle contraction and relaxation required for control. This therapy is typically performed by physical and occupational therapists.

BREATHWORK
Description and Mechanism of Action
Breathing connects the body with the environment, brings oxygen to the lungs and tissues, and influences neurologic control of automatic body functions. Breathwork simply means turning attention to the power and experience of the breath to improve relaxation, reduce stress, and "settle the mind."

Changes in breathing rate, rhythm, and volume serve as feedback signals to change nerve control of the autonomic nervous system. In other words, stress can cause fast breathing, which in turn signals the sympathetic nervous system to increase output, further preparing the body for stress. The opposite is true of slow rhythmic breathing. These changes are involuntary. As you have learned in previous chapters, the breath is also under voluntary control and can be used to regulate and switch gears from an overactive sympathetic nervous system or stress response to a parasympathetic nervous system or relaxation response. With practice and attention to breathing, the parasympathetic system can be enhanced and blood pressure, heart rate, anxiety, and muscle tension can improve.

"Direct and conscious breathing" differentiates breathwork from other forms of mind-body medicine. There are many different techniques and surely each one has benefits that can be tailored to the needs of individuals. General concepts shared by different techniques include the guided (self- or practitioner-guided) attention on breath with a focus on:

- Continuous and rhythmic rhythm
- Full active inhalation
- Relaxation and letting go through exhalation
- Combined use with mindfulness techniques or positive affirmation

Use in Parkinson's
There are no studies to date exploring the use of this technique for PD. Nonetheless, this technique can be especially helpful to calm the body and mind especially during times of anxiety or uncertainty. Breathwork is a practice, and with any practice it is easier to do over time. Examples of problems that breathwork can potentially help with are:

- Depression and anxiety
- Increased breath support and speech volume
- Stress management

- Sleep problems
- Muscle pain

Precautions

Breathing sustains life. As such, there should be few, if any, side effects. You may have trouble relaxing by focusing on the breath if you have symptoms of shortness of breath. Breathing problems can be caused by heart or lung disease. Breathing problems in PD can have multiple causes:

- Tightness, which you may experience in medicine off times due to rigidity of chest muscles
- Difficulty breathing due to restriction of air flow caused by flexed or slumped posture
- Respiratory dyskinesia, a problem of irregular breathing often experienced with medicine on time and visual signs of upper body dyskinesia

Breathing problems can cause anxiety, which further worsens sensation of shortness of breath. Although difficult in the beginning, the practice of calming and regulating your breathing can reduce the sense of anxiety that accompanies shortness of breath.

Guidance

Breathwork is free, easy to do, and can be done anywhere. Start by taking a few minutes each day to "check in" with your body and "tune into" the breath. Try the following simple method:

- Sit with your eyes gently closed or stand relaxed but with good posture, and focus on a distant object.
- Attend to your breathing by listening and feeling the breath in your body.
- Slowly breathe in by expanding the abdomen and the chest. Count from one to four (or less, if this is more comfortable), pause, and then slowly exhale, making a "whooshing" sound to a count that is slightly greater than the inhale. Focus simply on slowing and deepening the breath if this is uncomfortable or difficult.
- Repeat for a count of ten breaths.
- Open your eyes and simply take notice of how you feel. Take note of any good feelings or changes to reinforce the coupling of breath to feelings of well-being.

GUIDED IMAGERY

Description and Mechanism of Action

Guided imagery uses mental imagery for relaxation or to elicit a positive emotional state. Imagery is guided through verbal instruction or suggestions, visualization of a relaxing or positive image, or the use of music. A series of instructions or suggestions guides a person's internal images or visualizations toward relaxation or positive associations. This technique connects the visual and auditory brain circuits with emotional and cognitive circuits to influence thoughts and feelings. Guided imagery can be performed with a therapist, through the use of a CD or DVD, or with practice through self-guidance.

Use in Parkinson's

Guided imagery reduced tremor in people with PD after one brief session. In this study tremor severity was measured in 20 patients after 15-minute sessions of guided imagery, simple relaxation, and listening to relaxing music. Guided imagery had the most significant impact and longest effect on tremor with subjective effects lasting from one to 14 hours. This study is a powerful reminder that relaxation techniques can impact tremor. Of interest, guided imagery had better results than passive relaxation techniques. In a similar study, guided imagery also improved motor on time. Once again guided imagery was superior to relaxation by listening to music. Motor on time increased by 12% after three months of therapy. These findings are in line with other mind-body techniques showing enhanced brain activation when the experience is coupled with intentional focus of the mind.

(Refer also to the information on meditation and yoga nidra and its effect on brain dopamine, which is described later in this chapter.)

Precautions

Like many mind-body techniques, there are few contraindications. It is important to feel comfortable with the technique before starting. Be aware that each individual will have his or her own visual images that illicit well-being or even stress. Since this technique relies heavily on visual imagery, talk to your therapist about any images that you find pleasing or distressing. For instance, the image of water, the beach, and tides is calming but may be distressing if you are fearful of water or have had prior negative experiences associated with these images. If you are using a CD or DVD, simply start by listening. This will help you gauge whether the tone and voice of the person and the suggestions and images are best for you.

Guidance

Guided imagery is a good starting point for many interested in mind-body techniques yet not ready to attend a class or formal therapy. The guided or instructional nature of this therapy relieves the worries that you "just can't sit still and meditate" or concerns that "my mind is too scattered to focus," or "I don't have time," or "I am self-conscious about attending a class."

Many healing arts specialists including psychologists, yoga therapists, music and art therapists, massage therapists, and even chiropractors and physical therapists use guided imagery as part of their practice. The Academy for Guided Imagery (www.acadgi.com) has a professional training program for practitioners. The website www.healthjourneys.com offers many guided imagery products, including one specifically for PD.

HYPNOSIS

Description and Mechanism of Action

Hypnosis is described as a state of consciousness or a trance state. The desired result is focused attention, reduced distraction of thought, and enhanced response to suggestion. Brain studies suggest that specific brain areas are activated during hypnotic states. Different desired effects of hypnosis such as mental relaxation or mental attention are associated with different patterns of change in brain activity. Hypnosis is often done to reduce stress or reinforce a behavioral change such as weight loss or smoking cessation. People differ in the degree to which they respond to hypnosis, which may in part be related to beliefs about hypnosis.

A common misconception is that hypnosis is mind control. Just the opposite can be true. Awareness and control over thoughts and behavior are maintained and sometimes even sharpened. Hypnosis is performed while sitting or lying down in a comfortable state. The hypnotherapist then guides the individual through suggestions designed to enhance relaxation and work toward a predetermined goal.

Use in Parkinson's

Hypnosis is perhaps the earliest "modern" mind-body therapy to be studied in PD, with publications dating to the 1940s. Reports on the use of hypnosis for PD are limited to case studies showing improvement in tremor. One case report of an individual that used hypnosis for tremor control also reported improvements in anxiety, depression, sleep, libido, and quality of life. Hypnosis has been effectively used to change behaviors such as overeating, alcohol consumption, and smoking.

Because research in the use of hypnosis for PD is limited, observational studies from single individuals are sometimes used. Although illustrative and of potential benefit, observational studies do not have the scientific rigor needed to apply to the broader PD community. However, hypnosis does have strong evidence to support its use for stress management and relaxation, both of which will have positive benefits in PD.

Precautions

Hypnosis is used as a healing therapy by diverse clinicians and therapists trained in patient care. Unfortunately, hypnosis is also adopted by personal coaches, entertainers, and self-help promoters without appropriate training. If you are interested in hypnosis, be sure that your therapist is trained in both the technique and clinical management of any emotional issues that may present during or after hypnosis.

Guidance

Some states do not regulate the practice of hypnosis. Be sure that you are working with a practitioner who has appropriate training and experience in hypnosis, but also be aware that there is no unified training or qualification required to practice clinical hypnosis. Begin, then, by looking for a practitioner who carries a clinical license recognized by your state, such as a psychologist, physician, or clinical social worker. There are many professional organizations dedicated to the training and quality of hypnotherapy. The following organizations offer information on hypnosis, training, and certification:

- American Society of Clinical Hypnosis, www.asch.net
- National Board for Certified Clinical Hypnotherapists, www.natboard.com

MEDITATION AND MINDFULNESS

Description and Mechanism of Action

Meditation is a broad term defining many practices designed to focus the mind to enhance relaxation, gain insight and control over emotional and physical responses to daily experiences, and improve compassion and mental or physical performance. Meditation has its roots in spiritual and religious traditions and continues to be used within this context. Meditation practices are now an important part of many wellness and chronic disease programs.

Meditation can be performed both informally and formally. There are many formal practices, structured programs, and philosophical teachings available. Some of the guiding principles that underlie various forms of meditation are as follows:

- *Concentrative.* This form uses focus and the elimination of distraction to sharpen and strengthen the mind. Examples include Zen meditation and transcendental meditation (TM). In TM, a mantra (repeated word or phrase) is used to focus the mind and attention. Breath is used to alter states of mind.
- *Heart Centered.* The focus is on loving kindness and compassion toward one's self, others, and any other relationship such as the environment. This meditation serves to help eliminate negative thoughts, obstructions, and rigid thinking.
- *Mindfulness.* Bringing attention or awareness to the moment without judgment is the definition of mindfulness. Focus is on observation, insight, and letting go. Mindfulness is particularly helpful for living with chronic illness since it encourages living life to the fullest either despite, in response to, or as a result of difficulties. This is done through awareness of life's

overlooked moments and understanding that each moment is imper-manent, that change is a part of life and you have control of your mind's thoughts in the moment. This awareness can prevent the downward spiral of negative thinking that can accompany distress.

- *Reflective.* In this form of meditation the focus is on critical and focused think-ing. A question or theme is chosen to gain better clarity and understanding.

- *Creative and Visualization.* This form of meditation focuses on an event, activity, or desired goal.

Many of these principles are an integral part of therapies already reviewed, such as yoga, tai chi, qigong, and guided imagery. Mindfulness-Based Stress Reduc-tion® (MBSR) is a successful meditative practice promoted by medical practi-tioners to help people live with pain, anxiety, depression, fear, or symptoms of chronic illness. This eight-week program, founded by Dr. Jon Kabat-Zinn and colleagues at the University of Massachusetts, is now offered throughout the United States in many medical and community centers.

Brain research (too numerous to include in this book) shows improved brain activity, including an increase in brain size and positive neurochemical, immune, and hormonal activity, with meditation.

Use in Parkinson's

Studies examining the effect of meditation and mindfulness in PD are in their infancy. Mindfulness-based cognitive therapy can help coping skills and the sense of loss that can accompany change associated with PD. Although rigor-ous studies specific to PD are just beginning, studies of mindfulness meditation in people with other chronic conditions show improvements in the following symptoms:

- Levels of distress, coping, and adjustment
- Quality of life
- Depression, anxiety, sleep, fatigue, and pain
- Mental function

Meditation can change measures of brain activity and size. Increase in gray matter brain density was measured by MRI in the amygdala, hippocampus, thal-amus, and caudate nucleus (important brain structures for control of movement, learning, and stress) of people with PD. Of note, changes in amygdala volume are associated with PD-related anxiety. Mindfulness-based yoga nidra, a medi-tation technique often coupled with yoga practice, can change brain biochemis-try during practice. In this practice the body is relaxed in a sitting or lying position and the mind is intentionally allowed to drift in a sleeplike state but with full con-scious awareness. Yoga nidra is associated with increased dopamine levels in the striatum as measured by PET scan. Although subjects in this study did not have PD, it is of potential significance since the striatum and dopamine regulation is a significant part of PD neuropathology.

Precautions

There are few risks associated with meditation. Distress can come from paying attention to and increasing your awareness of thoughts and behaviors. Individuals with psychotic disorders, significant depression, or post-traumatic stress disorder should meditate under the care of a mental health professional.

Guidance

Look for a mindfulness-based therapy, class, or practitioner affiliated with your local medical center or hospital to ensure that the instructor is trained in applying these therapies to medical conditions. MBSR® is a standardized eight-week course taught by instructors who are often medical providers and have undergone specific training.

INTERVIEW WITH THE EXPERT: MINDFULNESS MEDITATION

Through mindfulness you come to realize you are not your illness

How did you get started in your work with mindfulness?

I was raised in the Christian tradition but exposed to other wisdom and devotional traditions from childhood, so meditation practices from various traditions—Buddhist, Christian, Jewish, Hindu—have always been part of my life. I started studying and practicing mindfulness formally in 1982 with teachers in the United States, Tibet, Nepal, and India, and have continued practice and study since then, and now live it in my personal and professional life.

How has living mindfully enriched your life?

Paraphrasing the poet, Rilke says, "When we come into the present moment, we awaken to the unbearable beauty within and around us, and the unspeakable pain of the world." Practicing mindfulness brings me in touch with the deep perennial wisdom and compassion that are always available within us, informing, guiding, and deeply enriching both my personal and professional life as a clinical and health psychologist practicing psychotherapy, conducting research, teaching in universities, and training lay people and professionals in mindfulness at Duke University Medical Center.

(continued)

INTERVIEW WITH THE EXPERT (*continued*)

How can this mindfulness potentially help people with PD?

What I have learned from my clients with PD—or virtually any state of disease in the body or mind—is that by practicing mindfulness, clients begin to live more mindfully, more fully, and more joyfully, with significantly greater resilience and resourcefulness. Through mindfulness, you come to realize that you are not your illness—not your symptoms, not reduced to the label of being a "PD patient or victim," not your thoughts, feelings, or stories about having PD or any other disease—but you are instead much more vast and boundless than any condition of the body/mind and any and all thoughts and feelings combined. Your identity and lives do not become limited to or restricted by the conditions of the body. [My clients] broaden and build resilience with mindfulness by becoming more aware of body sensations, thoughts, and feelings in a loving, accepting, skillfully responsive way, and learn how to wisely and lovingly work with them in optimally supportive and effective ways. That can mean learning to mindfully pace types and levels of activity and energy expenditure, mindfully exercising and engaging in healthy movement for your body, mindfully eating foods that are wholesome and nutritious for your body, mindfully getting appropriate levels of deep and restorative sleep, collaborating in a partnering way with health and mental health care providers for healing, and engaging with family, friends, and loved ones in mindful ways that support the journey together with PD as part of their lives. It can also mean mindfully discovering how to view PD as your teacher, friend, and ally: awaken and be open to the gifts of ever-deepening wisdom and compassion as a result of experiencing PD, recognizing your interconnectedness with all beings and things, held and supported by the boundless and loving vastness that is always within you and that we are all a part of and that is called by many names—spacious awareness, great mystery, and more. . . .

How is mindfulness-based meditation different from other forms of meditation?

In my experience, two of the most striking ways mindfulness is unique is that it includes a) the intentional practice of unconditional loving acceptance of self and all that is, and b) the awareness of the ever-changing, impermanent, interdependent nature of this relative

(*continued*)

INTERVIEW WITH THE EXPERT (*continued*)

world, which helps us loosen our tendency to grasp for and cling to that which we like and push away that which we dislike. This ultimately helps us reduce our and others' suffering in this world.

How can someone get started in the journey to live more mindfully?

There is an old Zen saying that goes something like, "That which is learned cannot be spoken." That is to say, in order to truly know something, one must experience it directly. For example, if you really want to know what love is, one has to experience it. So to really know what mindfulness is, we do it, not only read or talk about it. So, my best invitation is to take a mindfulness class or workshop, or attend a mindfulness retreat with a reputable teacher—preferably in person, on site. However, online opportunities can also be a helpful way to start, as many online programs provide access to teacher-led guidance. In addition, one can practice with DVDs or CDs and can augment practice by listening to talks about mindfulness and reading books. Duke has on-site courses, retreats, and other practice opportunities, along with distance-learning courses and course materials and CDs available for purchase if one cannot attend the in-person, on-site courses. This information can be found at www.dukeintegrativemedicine.org.

Maya McNeilly, PhD
Duke University Medical Center,
Department of Integrative Medicine

Dr. McNeilly is a licensed practicing clinical and health psychologist who teaches mindfulness, conducts research, and has a mindfulness-based private psychotherapy practice.

References

Biofeedback

Burgio, K. L., et al. 2002. "Behavioral training with or without biofeedback in the treatment of urge incontinence in older women." *JAMA* 288: 2293–99.

Breathwork

Lelande, L. 2011. "Breathwork: An additional treatment option for depression and anxiety?" *Journal of Contemporary Psychotherapy* 42: 113–19.

Guided Imagery

Schlesinger, I. 2009. "Parkinson's disease tremor is diminished with relaxation guided imagery." *Movement Disorders* 24: 2059–62.

————. 2014. "Relaxation guided imagery reduces motor fluctuations in Parkinson's disease." *Journal of Parkinson's Disease* 4: 431–36.

Hypnosis

Elkins, G., et al. 2013. "Feasibility of clinical hypnosis for the treatment of Parkinson's: A case study." *International Journal of Clinical Hypnosis* 61: 172–82.

Rainville, P., et al. 2002. "Hypnosis modulates activity in brain structures involved in the regulation of consciousness." *Journal of Cognitive Neuroscience* 14: 887–901.

Wain, H. J. 1990. "The effects of hypnosis on a parkinsonian tremor: Case report with polygraph/EEG recordings." *American Journal of Clinical Hypnosis* 33: 94–98.

Meditation and Mindfulness

Fitzpatrick, L. 2010. "A quantitative analysis of mindfulness-based cognitive therapy (MBCT) in Parkinson's." *Psychology and Psychotherapy: Theory, Research, and Practice* 83: 179–92.

Kabat- Zinn, J. 1990. *Full Catastrophe Living: Using the Wisdom of Your Body and Mind to Face Stress, Pain, and Illness.* New York: Delacourt.

Kiaer, T. W. 2002. "Increased dopamine tone during meditation-induced change of consciousness." *Cognitive Brain Research* 13: 255–59.

Pickutt, B. A., et al. 2013. "Mindfulness-based intervention in Parkinson's disease leads to structural changes in MRI: A randomized controlled longitudinal trial." *Clinical Neurology and Neurosurgery* 115: 2419–25.

Vriend, C., P. S. Boedhoe, S. Rutten, et al. 2015. "A smaller amygdala is associated with anxiety in Parkinson's disease: A combined FreeSurfer-VBM study." *Journal of Neurology, Neurosurgery, and Psychiatry.* doi:10.1136/jnnp-2015-310383

CHAPTER

9

Energy and Sensory Medicine

Energy medicine is based on the premise that energy is an important part of health and balance. Systems of energy exist within our body, between individuals, and in the environment. Balance of these energy systems affects health, and blockage or disequilibrium impacts disease. Energy comes in many forms and can be divided into veritable energy (measurable) and putative energy (not measurable).

Here's a simple example that illustrates how energy or an unmeasurable force affects outcome. Think about walking into a room, perhaps attending a social event. Think about how individuals in the room and the interactions (conversation, expression, body language) between people and even the room itself take on a certain energy. In this situation sights, sounds, and emotions culminate to create a sensation or perception (*a feeling*) of energy and change behavior.

Examples of energy forms that can promote healing include:

- Sound
- Visual
- Heat
- Electromechanical
- Tactile (touch)
- Emotional

Energy can be directly applied or experienced, as is the case of heat or sound, respectively. Practitioners of this field also believe that energy can be channeled from healer to recipient. There is little scientific research to support the use of these therapies to treat and heal. However, lack of information does not always mean lack of benefit. Some forms of energy are not as yet measurable; nonetheless, they are felt. As the previous example highlights, the sights and smells in a room, or even people in it, bring a certain energy to the room. As we explore these therapies, we will examine the proposed mechanisms for how they may work and, when appropriate, alternative theories for their benefit.

Many energy therapies are also sensory therapies as they activate our senses of sight, touch, taste, smell, and hearing. Aromatherapy is one example.

ACUPUNCTURE
Description and Mechanism of Action
Acupuncture is an ancient form of healing originating over 2,500 years ago and grounded in traditional Chinese medicine. Different forms or styles of acupuncture are performed in the United States, influenced by Chinese, Japanese, or Korean medicine. An acupuncturist inserts tiny needles into specific body areas to change the flow of energy or *Qi*. Health is associated with unobstructed energy flow, disease is associated with blocked Qi. Energy flows through the body along channels or meridians. There are 12 paired meridians that travel up and down both sides of the body and two unpaired meridians. Meridians are associated with specific organs in the body. Acupuncture points are locations where these meridians are close to the skin surface.

There are many different techniques and styles of acupuncture, including:

- *Needling:* insertion of different types of metal needles at different angles, force, vibration
- *Electroacupuncture:* application of a small amount of electricity to stimulate the area
- *Moxibustion:* applying heat
- *Cupping:* applying suction
- *Acupressure:* applying pressure
- *Reflexology:* applying pressure to the feet
- *Sonopuncture:* applying ultrasound
- *Auriculotherapy:* acupuncture applied to the ear

Acupuncture is gaining acceptance in Western medicine as an effective tool to help mood problems, nausea associated with chemotherapy, headache, and arthritic and muscular pain. Although not vigorously proven via the scientific method, acupuncture has improved pain and short-term tremor control for some people with Parkinson's disease (PD).

Animal studies are showing potential acupuncture benefits on brain activity and cellular changes associated with PD pathology. Research findings (measured in rodents not people) indicate certain brain changes caused by acupuncture. For example, acupuncture:

- Prevents dopamine nerve cell damage caused by inflammation or neuro-toxin injection in animals
- Increases dopamine release and movement in animal models of PD
- Increases nerve cell protective antioxidant activity in nerve cells of animals
- Increases activity in the frontal lobes (responsible for emotional and cognitive function)

Of interest, acupuncture stimulation of the point GB34 activates neural responses associated with PD.

Use in Parkinson's

Acupuncture is the most studied energy therapy in PD. Prior studies were predominantly without placebo, but newer studies are placebo-controlled to truly test the effect of therapy vs. placebo. Open label studies (no placebo, all participants receiving acupuncture) did reveal improvements or trends toward improved sleep, finger tapping movements, and quality of life. One study analyzing the effect of acupuncture on brain activity in 12 people with PD showed increased activity as measured by functional MRI in key regions of the basal ganglia in PD. The open label nature of this study, however, could not prove that these changes were specific to acupuncture itself.

Perhaps some of the strongest evidence in support of acupuncture is in the control of neck and back pain. Back and neck pain is common in PD and this therapy is yet another avenue of treatment that can complement traditional pain management.

Precautions

Acupuncture is not for everyone. In general, its use for pain control is associated with the strongest evidence. This may be due to the possibility that pain is best treated with acupuncture and/or is the most commonly or easiest to study. As always, be sure that your therapist has the training and experience with your condition. Be wary of a therapist that insists on long-term therapy without clear benefit.

There are many different types of acupuncture including electroacupuncture and acupressure. Also many acupuncture sessions combine other therapies, such as counseling, music, relaxation, or aromatherapy. Therefore, it is very difficult to understand true acupuncture outcomes given the many ways it is done, accompanying therapies that are used with it, and the differences in acupuncture training ranging from brief courses to doctoral level training. Deep brain stimulation (DBS) wires are coiled under the scalp and are not easy to palpate. Piercing DBS wires with an acupuncture needle will damage the wire. For this reason, acupuncture is not recommend over the scalp, neck, or upper chest if you have DBS.

Guidance

Acupuncture is performed individually or in a group setting. Be sure to talk to your acupuncturist about your goals (e.g., sleep, pain, tremor, or mood) and about how many treatments should be tried before determination of effect. This prevents a situation in which you continue to get therapy (and spend the money) that is not effective over a long period of time.

Like all healing arts, be sure you know how your acupuncturist is trained and whether the practitioner is certified to perform this therapy. An acupuncturist can be a medical doctor but can also be a non-physician. Some acupuncturists have training and doctoral degrees in Chinese medicine. The National Certification Commission for Acupuncture and Oriental Medicine (NCCAOM, www.nccaom .org) offers an examination to practitioners to ensure minimal competency. Most states require that clinicians are licensed to provide acupuncture. Visit the American Association of Acupuncture and Oriental Medicine (AAAOM, www.aaao monline.org) for more information.

AROMATHERAPY
Description and Mechanism of Action

Aromatherapy is the use of essential oils to impact health and healing either through inhalation or application to the skin. Essential oils are extracted from plants. These essential oils or aromatic compounds isolated from plants are lipid (fat) soluble, which means they can be absorbed through the skin and the blood-brain barrier. The blood-brain barrier surrounds the brain and serves to filter chemicals and toxins from entrance into the brain. Two ways in which aromatherapy may work is through the direct action of the chemicals on brain receptors and through their influence on key brain structures designed to interpret smells. Smell is actually a complex sense and one deeply tied to our emotional state. Smell is an important sense used to connect us to our environment. The olfactory bulb (a collection of nerve cells in the nose) is directly connected to the primitive or emotional part of the brain called the limbic system. The limbic system registers smells and in turn sends neural connections to the frontal cortex, hippocampus, and hypothalamic regions. This complex neural network allows you to connect smell or aromas in the following ways:

- *Limbic System:* The primitive brain can influence your emotions, registering safety, danger, or distress. Smells or aromas send important chemical signals to influence mood or action. For instance, certain smells send warnings of danger or fear (toxins, decay) or pleasure (chocolate, flowers).
- *Hippocampus:* Part of the limbic system, the hippocampus is important in the processing of memories. In this way smells can be remembered along

with certain associated behaviors or feelings. For example, think of the powerful memories elicited by the smell of a loved one's perfume or the childhood memories that might be elicited with the smell of baking cookies.

- *Frontal Cortex:* The frontal cortex or our thinking brain can interpret primitive emotions and associated memories within the context of the current situation. For instance, the smell of chocolate chip cookies not only evokes memories of childhood but also the ideas of comfort and security, if these feelings were associated with those earlier times.

Aromatherapy is based on the chemical excitation of these neural pathways. Some aromas such as lavender and lemon balm increase neurotransmitters important for relaxation such as gamma-amino butyric acid (GABA). Others such as eucalyptus and peppermint increase norepinephrine and as a result can help energize, improve attention or focus. Essential oils also have strong antioxidant properties as measured by the Oxygen Radical Absorbance Capacity (ORAC) test. ORAC is a test developed by the U.S. Department of Agriculture and Tufts University to measure the antioxidant and free radical squelching capabilities of compounds.

Use in Parkinson's

Some of the earliest nerve changes in PD involve the olfactory bulb. Reduced or loss of smell can occur years before the first motor symptoms of PD. Even when smell is decreased, there may still be the ability to identify certain aromas. Certain smells are preferentially lost. Wintergreen and pizza (oregano) are odors most likely to be misidentified by people with PD. Without the sense of smell it is still possible that certain aromas can react chemically with key brain structures to trigger memories or evoke emotions.

There is limited evidence in support of aromatherapy for PD. A non-controlled study of aromatherapy with or without massage did show benefits. Whether these benefits are truly secondary to aromatherapy are not clear. Aromatherapy is often used to calm and reduce agitation in dementia. Loss of smell is often associated with dementia as well as PD. A review of multiple studies investigating the use of aromatherapy in dementia were equivocal.

Precautions

Aromatherapy oils are concentrated essential oils that are plant derived. Certain oils can be irritating to skin and toxic if ingested.

Not every person with PD has complete loss of smell. You can experiment with your ability to register certain smells that may evoke strong positive memories or sensations such as:

- *Alertness:* coffee, peppermint, eucalyptus
- *Stress relief and relaxation:* lemon balm, lavender
- *Emotional well-being:* chocolate, cinnamon

If you can register the smell, there are many ways you can use it for the desired effect. Examples include use of candles, potpourri, essential oil added to eye or neck pillows, and bath creams or lotions. You can learn more about aromatherapy through the National Association for Holistic Aromatherapy (NAHA, www.naha.org).

HEALING OR THERAPEUTIC TOUCH

Description and Mechanism of Action

Healing touch is a form of energy medicine in which practitioners use their hands in a heart-centered way to heal. This technique was founded by a nurse, Janet Mentgen, in 1989 and derived from her observations of the healing power of touch and the therapeutic relationship between nurse and patient. According to the Healing Touch Program™ (www.healingtouchprogram.com), this therapy uses the practitioner's hands to balance and restore the energy field that surrounds the body. Each session consists of the practitioner placing hands over the body without touching to read energy fields and restore energy balance.

Sessions are conducted much in the same way massage is performed, in a calm and relaxing environment often coupled with comforting music or sounds.

Use in Parkinson's

Healing touch is reported to help many conditions and symptoms including stress, pain, and immune function. Many studies supporting benefits exist, but very few offer quality information supportive of these claims.

Precautions

There is no evidence for benefit in PD. Risk is minimal.

Guidance

Proposed benefits for healing touch are largely anecdotal and based on personal experiences. Whether improvements are secondary to the specific treatment itself or other healing factors is not certain. The relaxing environment, healing expectations of the recipient, compassionate nature of the practitioner, and the caring therapeutic relationship between patient and practitioner are just some of the nonspecific ways that healing touch can reduce stress, enhance well-being, and improve mood and symptoms such as pain and muscle spasm. Healing touch is associated with low risk as long as you are aware that benefits may be related to these other factors and not necessarily the therapy itself. This is important to understand before you begin a healing touch session. Be wary of reports claiming dramatic results, cures, or requiring extensive and expensive sessions. Training does exist for healing touch practitioners.

LIGHT THERAPY

Description and Mechanism of Action

Light therapy uses natural daylight or artificial light designed to simulate natural sunlight. Light reacts with cells in the retina to reset circadian rhythms. Circadian rhythms, otherwise known as your internal biological clock, regulate 24-hour cycles such as sleep and wakefulness. Light therapy is used to normalize the sleep-wake cycle and treat seasonal or winter depression. Research suggests that light therapy can phase-shift or advance circadian rhythms and block the release of melatonin, a natural neurohormone that influences sleep onset.

Bright light benefits may extend beyond seasonal depression to include major depression unrelated to the season.

Use in Parkinson's

Depression is common, affecting up to half of people with PD. Additional and perhaps more common symptoms are daytime fatigue and night-time sleep problems. Emerging evidence suggests bright light therapy may be useful to treat these problems. One hypothesis is that those with PD (and the elderly) can suffer from phase advance in their circadian rhythms (early to bed and early to rise), which can disrupt sleep and other symptoms such as mood and daytime alertness. Studies evaluating the effect of bright light therapy are small but do suggest a modest benefit. In particular, a controlled trial of people receiving 15-day, 30-minute daily, 7,500-lux[1] light therapy showed improvement in mood, sleep, activities, and tremor. Although not tested for PD dementia, bright light coupled with melatonin may also reduce cognitive decline associated with dementia.

Precautions

Bright light may not be safe for everyone and should be used with caution if you have certain skin and eye conditions that are associated with photosensitivity, such as porphyria, lupus, macular degeneration, and certain retinal disease. Certain medicines such as tricyclic antidepressants and antibiotics such as tetracycline cause skin sensitivity to light and interact with this therapy. Bright light side effects include increased eyestrain, headache, agitation, and mania in people with bipolar disorder. Discuss the use of bright light with your dermatologist, ophthalmologist, or primary physician before starting.

Guidance

It is not clear whether light therapy is best used in the morning (commonly prescribed for depression) or evening (to delay sleep onset and awakening) in PD. Typical light intensity ranges from 5,000 to 10,000 lux and the duration of therapy

---

[1] One lux is equivalent to the illumination of one candle.

is usually 15 to 45 minutes. Avoid light in the blue spectrum and look for a light with an ultraviolet (UV) filter since these wavelengths can cause skin and eye (retina) damage. Sit in front of the light source placed an arm's length away, but do not stare or look directly into the light. A light visor is also available for this purpose.

People with PD have an increased risk of melanoma, a serious form of skin cancer. Consider including a dermatologist as part of your medical team. This specialist can help you understand the risk of light therapy prior to its use and perform screening examinations to identify skin lesions suspicious for this malignant cancer.

MAGNET THERAPY

Description and Mechanism of Action

Small static (non-pulsing) magnets such as those found in bracelets are marketed for control of pain, reduced inflammation, and tissue healing. How magnets might work is not clear. At least one study in rodents did show measurable changes in blood vessel dilation, which potentially leads to improved blood flow, tissue oxygenation, and nutrient supply to damaged tissue and reduced inflammation caused by tissue damage. Effects in people are controversial, with conflicting study results and little support for benefit in controlled studies.

Transcranial magnetic stimulation (TMS) is distinct from small wearable magnets and is a medical procedure in which a special coil is placed on the scalp over specific brain areas. Pulsed stimulation penetrates through tissue and stimulates adjacent brain tissue. Stimulation of the frontal cortex can improve symptoms of major depression when delivered five times a week for four to six weeks. This therapy is now approved by the Food and Drug Administration (FDA) for major depression.

Use in Parkinson's

There is no evidence to support the use of static magnets for motor symptoms, pain, or inflammation. For treatment of depression associated with PD, of interest is a study that analyzed the effect of TMS vs. the antidepressant fluoxetine (Paxil®). The study measured a similar antidepressant effect for the two treatments but noted fewer side effects from TMS and a trend toward earlier improvement in cognitive function.

Precautions

Magnets of any kind placed on the body may not be safe if you have a pacemaker, DBS implant, insulin pump, or other electronic device since the magnetic field can interfere with the function of these devices. TMS is FDA approved only for major depression refractory or resistant to medications and must be performed by psychiatrists or other physicians trained in this therapy. Side effects do exist, including head and facial pain, muscle twitching, and seizure.

Guidance

Research using TMS is in its infancy and may show future promise; however, there is no support for use of magnets or TMS at this time. Also, TMS is not without risk, including the risk of seizure.

REIKI

Description and Mechanism of Action

Reiki is a Japanese technique for healing and stress reduction that works on the premise that an unseen energy or life force flows within our bodies and between individuals. Through placement of hands on different areas of the body, the Reiki practitioner is able to transfer, guide, and direct flow of energy.

Use in Parkinson's

Like many mind-body therapies there are no objective controlled studies evaluating the effect of Reiki on PD, and benefits rely on personal stories and experiences. Nonetheless, Reiki is a therapy that can result in healing, well-being, and stress management. It is unknown if benefits are specific to the technique or secondary to the healing abilities of the practitioner and the healing environment in which it is practiced.

Meta-analysis of multiple studies do suggest that Reiki may have positive effects on pain and anxiety.

Precautions

There is no evidence for benefit in PD. Risk is minimal.

Guidance

Reiki benefits are largely anecdotal and based on personal experiences. Whether improvements are secondary to the specific treatment itself or other healing factors is not certain. The relaxing environment, healing expectations of the recipient, compassionate nature of the practitioner, and the caring therapeutic relationship between patient and practitioner are just some of the nonspecific ways that Reiki can reduce stress, enhance well-being, and improve symptoms such as pain, mood, and muscle spasm. Reiki is associated with low risk as long as you are aware that benefits may be related to these other factors and not necessarily the therapy itself. This is important to understand before you begin a Reiki session. Be wary of reports claiming dramatic results, cures, or requiring extensive and expensive sessions. Training and certification does exist for Reiki practitioners. A Master Reiki practitioner has a reached higher level of training. You can also learn to perform Reiki on yourself, which can be helpful during times of stress, anxiety, problems with motor control, or pain.

INTERVIEW WITH THE EXPERT: REIKI

A HUSBAND AND WIFE TEAM BRING COMPASSION AND HEALING TO THE PARKINSON'S COMMUNITY

How did you get started in your work with Reiki?

I was not looking for Reiki, but Reiki found me. Seven years after my diagnosis with young onset PD, on a recommendation from someone I trusted, I investigated a modality called Trager and made contact with a local practitioner. The local practitioner was Gilbert Gallego, who was also a Reiki Master and incorporated other healing modalities. I remember Gallego telling me prior to my first session with him that he did Reiki, which involved "universal life-force *energy*." I had gone for something different [Trager] and was now exposed to Reiki, which I knew nothing about. My skepticism came from not knowing and having never heard of or experienced Reiki. I strongly considered leaving his office without trying it. I was having a bad day of PD symptoms, such as poor gait, stiffness, and low energy. I surmised as long as I was there, I didn't have that much to lose. I was so glad that I stayed.

Once his hands lightly touched my shoulders, I fell into a deep refreshing slumber. I awoke about an hour later feeling restored and refreshed. I did not know what it was or how it worked, but I knew my body needed more of whatever this was. I was hooked!

Initially, my wife Angela and I studied Reiki to help ourselves and improve our own self-care. We took our Reiki First Degree training in 1999, Second Degree in 2001, and Third Degree in 2004. It was never our intention to teach Reiki or work on other people. In 2008, we decided to introduce Reiki to the PD community by creating First Degree classes for people with PD and their care partners/caregivers. By introducing these two communities of people to each other, we realized that it would beneficial if we became Reiki Masters so that we could teach Reiki. In 2012, we completed a yearlong mastership program to educate and inform the PD community about the benefits of Reiki.

How can this therapy potentially help people with Parkinson's?

As each person with PD is unique, so are the benefits from Reiki. From my personal experience, Reiki helps me fall asleep, it lowers my stress and helps me center myself. Reiki can stop or nearly control my tremor

(*continued*)

INTERVIEW WITH THE EXPERT (*continued*)

and dyskinesia. Reiki has provided me some relief from my PD symptoms and taught me how to mentally cope with the daily surprises of the
illness. Reiki has brought me peace, control, and strength. Sixteen years
ago, I found Reiki as a skeptic, but when I discovered the tremendous
benefits of calmness and energy that it has brought me, I knew this was
just what I needed. I have no doubt that Reiki is one of the key tools to
my success. As a Reiki practitioner and Reiki Master, I can tell you that I
have seen a change of some sort in every person that I have worked on.

What would a participant expect during sessions?

You may be asked to discuss what is happening in your life. The
practitioner will assist the client onto a massage table or chair. The
client is fully clothed, then is covered with a sheet or blanket. During
the treatment, the practitioner will lightly touch the client on the head,
neck, arms, torso, legs, and feet. The practitioner may also slide their
hands under the client's neck, shoulders, or back. Sessions can last from
45 minutes to an hour. Clients may experience a variety of physical
sensations. Clients may feel warmth/cold, tingling, waves of energy, or a
client may not feel anything at all. Clients may also fall asleep. Reiki
energy has an innate ability to go where the body needs energy.

How is Reiki different from other energy therapies?

Reiki can be different from other energy therapies because it involves
light touch on the energy centers of the body. Reiki also works on
multiple levels of the body.

How do you find a practitioner? What special certification or training should an instructor have?

It is so important to find a Reiki practitioner that you can connect with
and who will listen to your needs. Like any service provider, investigating and uncovering the right provider/practitioner may take a little work.
One of the best ways to find a practitioner is through a referral from
someone you trust. If you want to learn Reiki, an instructor in Reiki
should be a Reiki Master. There are many types of Reiki. We practice
Reiki Jin Kei Do. Reiki mastership varies according to the lineage. Find
instructors who have been practicing Reiki for a number of years and
have a personal Reiki practice that they work on themselves each day.

(*continued*)

INTERVIEW WITH THE EXPERT (*continued*)

Currently, there is no national or international certification organization for Reiki practitioners. Check with your local municipality to see if Reiki practitioners need to be licensed in your area.

The first level or degree of Reiki teaches us to do Reiki on ourselves. We would encourage everyone to take a First Degree class. First Degree Reiki is a wonderful way to care for yourself.

> *Karl Robb, Reiki Jin Kei Do Master*
> *Author of* A Soft Voice in a Noisy World: A Guide to Dealing
> and Healing with Parkinson's Disease

Mr. Robb has been living with PD for over 30 years. His wife Angela is also a Reiki professional.

WHOLE BODY VIBRATION THERAPY

Description and Mechanism of Action

Vibration therapy applies controlled low-frequency and low-amplitude vibration to body tissue. Whole body vibration is often applied while sitting in a chair or standing on a platform. Mechanical vibration stimulates the musculoskeletal system to react to these mechanical pulses. The pulses cause rapid contraction of muscle, changing position and stretch on tendons, ligaments, and joints. These quick reactive mechanical changes of the musculoskeletal system also activate important nerve structures responsible for movement, including parts of the sensory, vestibular, and balance nervous system.

Vibrational therapy units can be found in the community gym and are used as part of physical therapy. The movement of these units are very different in that gym machines often vibrate up and down in a vertical plane. The upward movement increases the effect of gravity on muscles, which is used to increase muscle strength. Vibration platform units used in physical therapy pivot side to side to stimulate reactive body changes important for balance. Different frequencies and amplitudes are used for each system.

Vibration therapy is also used to treat restless legs syndrome (RLS). This therapy and other treatments for RLS are reviewed in Chapter 13.

Use in Parkinson's

Results of research analyzing the effect of whole body vibration on motor performance in PD varies from no benefit to improved balance. These discrepancies are in part due to the fact that many different research paradigms, devices, frequencies, and protocols have been tested. One study showed improvement in balance but no difference between vibration therapy and conventional physical therapy.

Precautions
High-frequency units used in many gyms can cause muscle and joint injury, pain, and falls. Use only under the guidance of a physical therapist trained in the application of this therapy.

Guidance
Although the use of vibration platforms is appealing, experience confirms that improvement in balance and motor performance is best achieved through active and dynamic movement and exercise. If used, vibration therapy guided by a therapist should complement but not take the place of movement and exercise. There are a variety of personal trainers, coaches, and exercise specialists that offer programs targeted at PD. Begin first with a physical therapist trained in neurorehabilitation since therapy targeting balance, posture, and walking is so important to PD individuals (and aging).

References

Acupuncture

Cristian, A., et al. 2005. "Evaluation of acupuncture in the treatment of Parkinson's disease: A double-blind pilot study." *Movement Disorders* 20: 1185–88.

Lam, Y. C. 2008. "Efficacy and safety of acupuncture for idiopathic Parkinson's disease: A systemic review." *Journal of Alternative and Complementary Medicine* 14: 663–71.

Lee, M. S., et al. 2008. "Effectiveness of acupuncture of Parkinson's disease: A systemic review." *Movement Disorders* 23: 1505–11.

Liu, X. Y. 2004. "Electro-acupuncture stimulation protects dopaminergic neurons from inflammation-mediated damage in medial forebrain bundle-transected rats." *Experimental Neurology* 189: 189–96.

Seum-Nam, K., et al. 2011. "Acupuncture enhances the synaptic dopamine availability to improve motor function in a mouse model of Parkinson's disease." *PLoS One* 6: e27566. doi:10.1371/journal.pone.0027566

Wang, H. 2011. "The antioxidative effect of electro-acupuncture in a mouse model of Parkinson's disease." *PLoS One* 6: e19790. doi:10.1371/journal.pone.0019790

Yang, J. L., et al. 2011. "Neuroprotection effects of retained acupuncture in neurotoxin-induced Parkinson's disease mice." *Brain Behavior Immunity* 25: 1452–59.

Yeo, S., et al. 2014. "Acupuncture on GB34 activates the precentral gyrus and prefrontal cortex in Parkinson's." *BMC Complementary and Alternative Medicine* 14: 336.

Zeng, B. Y., et al. 2013. "Current development of acupuncture in Parkinson's disease." *International Review of Neurobiology* 111: 141–58.

Aromatherapy

Forrester, L. T. 2014. "Aromatherapy for dementia." *Cochrane Database of Systematic Reviews* 2: CD003150. doi:10.1002/14651858.CD003150.pub2

Hawkes, C. H., et al. 1999. "Is Parkinson's disease a primary olfactory disorder?" *Quarterly Journal of Medicine* 92: 473–80.

Price, S. 1996. "Parkinson's Disease Project." *Positive Health Online: Integrative Medicine for the 21st Century.* http://www.positivehealth.com/article/aromatherapy/parkinson-s-disease-project

Healing or Therapeutic Touch

Hammerschlag, R., B. L. Marx, and M. Aickin. 2014. "Nontouch biofield therapy: A systematic review of human randomized controlled trials reporting use of only nonphysical contact treatment." *Journal of Alternative and Complementary Medicine* 20: 881–92.

Light Therapy

Paus, S., et al. 2007. "Bright light therapy in Parkinson's disease: A pilot study." *Movement Disorders* 22: 1495–98.

Riemersma-van der Lek, R. F., et al. 2008. "Effect of bright light and melatonin on cognitive and noncognitive function in elderly residents of group care facilities: A randomized controlled trial." *Journal of American Medical Association* 299: 2642–55.

Magnet Therapy

Fregni, F., et al. 2004. "Repetitive transcranial magnetic stimulation is as effective as fluoxetine in the treatment of depression in patients with Parkinson's disease." *Journal of Neurology, Neurosurgery, and Psychiatry* 75: 1171–74.

Morris, C. E., and T. C. Skalak. 2008. "Acute exposure to a moderate strength static magnetic field reduces edema formation in rats." *American Journal of Physiology Heart and Circulatory Physiology* 294: H50–7.

O'Reardon, J. P., et al. 2007. "Efficacy and safety of transcranial magnetic stimulation in the acute treatment of major depression: A multisite randomized controlled trial." *Biological Psychiatry* 62: 1208–16.

Reiki

Thran, S., and S. M. Cohen. 2014. "Effect of Reiki therapy on pain and anxiety in adults: An in-depth literature review of randomized trials with effect size calculations." *Pain Management Nursing* 15: 897–908.

Whole Body Vibration Therapy

Ebersbach, G., et al. 2008. "Whole body vibration versus conventional physiotherapy to improve balance and gait in Parkinson's disease." *Archives of Physical Medicine and Rehabilitation* 89: 399–403.

CHAPTER

10

Community, Spirituality, Expressive, and Experiential Healing

This section reviews the healing arts that strengthen the spirit, expand horizons of thought, increase a sense of confidence or capability, add meaning to life, and strengthen connections to people and community. Some therapies that fall in this category—such as music therapy, healing and therapeutic touch, loving kindness, and mindfulness meditation—have been reviewed in prior chapters.

We often discuss holistic care as that which integrates the mind, body, and spirit. Most of you understand what we mean when we talk about the physical body. You understand, too, that the mind is synonymous with the ability to think and perhaps even our mood. But what is the spirit?

Our spirit lies at the very core of who we are,
what we cherish and hold true, and what we do.

There is not a single definition for the spirit or spirituality, since the essence of the spirit is personal and will mean different things to different people. There are, however, overriding themes that will resonate with each of you and that can help you through your life journey when suffering and disease threaten your sense of well-being.

Spirituality is personal. Some find spirituality through connection with religion, while others find spirituality in their connections with nature, the arts, and humanity. Spirituality can be connection with faith, a higher power, or the collective good. It embraces interconnectedness with family, friends, community, society, service, and the world. It is the power and importance of our ideas, values, and beliefs. Spirituality can be described as a meaningful purpose in life.

Healing and spirituality is of critical importance for people with Parkinson's disease (PD) since it connects personal suffering with personal meaning or values to heal. One can achieve a sense of wholeness beyond the physical self by embracing and supporting the spiritual self.

Our spiritual identity can be broken down into the following areas:

- *Thoughts:* Our thoughts include questions about meaning, what is important, and what gives purpose to life. As a person with PD, you may be thinking, *how do I continue along my life's path, start over, or change my life path?*

- *Feelings:* We experience emotions such as love, connection, community, hope, inner peace, joy, sorrow, desire, empathy, acceptance, and forgiveness. As a person with PD, *do these emotions hold true, and do they gain even stronger meaning and commitment?*

- *Actions:* We have relationships and interactions with others. Our actions include our commitment to church or organization, prayer and meditation, generosity in giving and support, and the very act of caring for ourselves and others. As a person with PD, you may wonder, *are there new ways to care for myself or others, new activities, priorities, relationships, or connections to make?*

The following resources can help you learn more about your own community and spiritual programs.

- *Local foundations*
- *Churches and religious groups*
- *Libraries*
- *Community and senior centers and park and recreation centers*
- *Community colleges*
- *Medical centers*

INTERVIEW WITH THE EXPERT: DANCE FOR PD®

THE POWER OF POSSIBILITY EXEMPLIFIED IN A COMMUNITY PARTNERSHIP PROGRAM

Dance for PD® is not about managing PD— for many participants it is an escape from PD.

How did you get started in your work with dance for Parkinson's?

Dance for PD®, is an innovative global program that has launched in more than 100 communities in 12 countries. This program began in 2001, when Olie Westheimer, the founder and executive director of the Brooklyn Parkinson Group (BPG), approached the Mark Morris Dance Group (MMDG), an internationally acclaimed modern dance company that had just opened a new dance center in Brooklyn. Westheimer proposed the idea of a rigorous, creative dance class for members of her group. That year, John Heginbotham and I—as dancers from the MMDG—along with a professional musician, began leading free monthly classes for a small group of people. A third dancer, Misty Owens, joined the teaching team shortly thereafter. Since the Dance for PD program is built on one fundamental premise—professionally trained dancers are movement experts whose knowledge is useful to persons with PD—the program's content and structure was developed by the dance instructors, in consultation with Westheimer and members of BPG.

How can this program potentially help people with Parkinson's?

The fundamentals of dancing and dance training—things like balance, movement sequencing, rhythm, spatial and aesthetic awareness, and dynamic coordination—seem to address many of the goals people with PD want to work on to maintain or improve their mobility. Because Dance for PD focuses on the aesthetic movement of dance rather than therapy, participants in the class are encouraged to approach movement like dancers rather than patients. By design, the class exists outside the traditional parameters of physical therapy and clinical rehabilitation.

(continued)

INTERVIEW WITH THE EXPERT (*continued*)

Dance for PD classes provide a close-knit social environment for participants to interact with other community members and to share a positive, stimulating activity together with their partners. Participants report, both anecdotally and as measured in preliminary studies, that the classes boost their confidence levels, combat social isolation and depression, transform their attitudes about living with a chronic illness, and help them manage some of the symptoms associated with PD.

What would a participant expect during sessions?

Classes, which last about 75 minutes, start with a seated, progressive dance warm-up, followed by supported standing activities at a chair or ballet bar. Classes finish with across-the-floor combinations that build on previous material. Dance for PD teaching artists integrate movement from modern and theater dance, ballet, folk dance, tap, improvisation, and choreographic repertory. All exercises can be done seated or standing so that people of all levels of ability and mobility can participate fully in the class. Teachers are trained to translate dance material for a wide range of participants. Everything is performed to live or recorded music.

How is Dance for PD different from other movement or exercise classes?

Dance is certainly good exercise, and movements are contemplative like yoga, but our class emphasizes the imaginative, creative, musical, expressive, social, and narrative elements that form that basis of dance as an art form. Participants use their imaginations in the service of dynamic, varied, expressive movement—and the goals of our class are aesthetic rather than therapeutic. Dance for PD is not about managing PD—for many participants it is an escape from PD. And yet every skill that a dancer thinks about and practices is beneficial for a person with a movement disorder. When we're dancing a scene from *West Side Story*, for example, we are working on balance, amplitude, facial expression, and rhythm. But we get at those things through the back door. The main focus is playing Sharks or Jets, practicing the choreography, and expressing elements of the story.

(*continued*)

INTERVIEW WITH THE EXPERT (continued)

How does one find a program?

Programs are listed and updated regularly on our website: www
.danceforpd.org. We regularly work to support individuals and groups
who want to start a class in their communities. We offer at-home
instructional DVDs for people who can't find a class near them.

What have you and your dancers and others learned about themselves by participating?

I've learned to reveal and celebrate the wide range of creative movement possibilities that exist in all human beings. Together, participants and I have learned about an incredible cycle: dancing together
creates community, and the social bonds within that community in
turn help to sustain the motivation to dance even when personal
circumstances become more challenging. Participants have learned
to value themselves more and to build a sense of hope, creativity,
and community into their daily lives. This focus on exploration and
possibility, rather than limitation, carries over into other activities
and relationships.

What special certification or training do instructors have?

All the instructors in our network have completed an introductory
training workshop with us, but almost all have already been teaching
dance for many years and have strong training in at least one dance
form. A Dance for PD certification program is available for those
teachers who have led an established class for several years and whose
teaching work and qualifications are of the highest standard.

David Leventhal, Program Director, Dance for PD®
Mark Morris Dance Group, danceforparkinsons.org

ANIMAL THERAPY AND SERVICE DOGS

Description and Mechanism of Action

Animal or pet therapy capitalizes on the strong positive emotional bond that
develops between people and animals to improve emotional well-being, confidence, independence, and strength. Service dogs are specially trained to help and
protect people with vision, hearing, physical, and emotional challenges. The

earliest and best-known use of service dogs is the use of guide dogs for blind or visually challenged persons. Animal therapy is the use of animals in a rehabilitative setting such as physical or occupational therapy.

The therapeutic potential of animal-assisted therapy is in part based on the theory of biophilia. This theory suggests that the strong connection and attachment between animals and people originated because people depended on signals from animals as clues about the safety or threats in an environment, necessary observations for survival. This developmental relationship explains why a friendly, playful, or resting animal conveys feelings of safety, protection, well-being, or connectedness.

Cats, dogs, and horses are the most common animals used for pet therapy or as service animals. The primary goals of animal-assisted therapy are to improve:

- Mobility and physical independence
- Socialization
- Emotional well-being
- Activity and community engagement

Use in Parkinson's

Animals are used to engage people and reduce loneliness, sadness, aggression, and agitation in nursing home residents. Service dogs can help a person with PD in many ways. The majority of people use a Mobility Assistance Dog to improve daily activities. As examples, a service dog may:

- Help with physical tasks around the house, such as turning on light switches, opening and closing doors, picking up objects.
- Assist with walking by helping with balance, acting as a support, or helping a person get up.
- Hold a person up if he or she gets dizzy.
- Overcome freezing of gait, which is accomplished by the dog clearing the way in crowded areas, by using gentle pressure on a person's leg, or leading a person away from a hectic and stressful area that can exacerbate freezing.
- Exert a calming effect at times of stress and anxiety.
- Pull objects such as the person's wheelchair, which is accomplished with the aid of a special harness worn by a Mobility Assistance Dog.

Examples of ways therapy animals support social and emotional well-being include:

- Improve mood, anxiety, and stress levels
- Increase self-confidence
- Enhance socialization
- Enhance motivation and engagement in life activity
- Reduce agitation associated with confusion, change, and new surroundings

Precautions

Risks associated with animal therapy go beyond concerns of animal allergy, cleanliness, and bites. Prior animal experiences can trigger anxiety or fear with certain animals. Physical assistance animals must be well trained. For example, animals that are not well trained could cause a fall rather than prevent a fall. It is best to leave this training to specialists and foundations focused on this mission.

Guidance

The following websites are sources of information about service animals:

- *Assistance Dogs International*, www.assistancedogsinternational.org, offers information on service dogs and answers to frequently asked questions.
- *Paws with a Cause*, www.pawswithacause.org/what-we-do/service-dogs, offers general information on service animals.

JOURNALING AND GRATITUDE
Description and Mechanism of Action

Journaling encourages daily reflection and is an effective exercise for personal development. Keeping a journal means that you will write (or record) a daily record of your experience. Caregivers, patients, and truly all of us can benefit from keeping a journal, which is different from a diary that focuses on daily activities or what you did for the day. This is an important part of journaling, but journaling includes much more.

Journaling can help you see the positive and the possibilities, and manage the difficult times and uncertainties about the future. Maintaining a sense of gratitude is an important focus of journaling. The word "gratitude" comes from the Latin root *gradia*, meaning gratefulness or grace. Gratitude is not easy to define but generally is a quality, action, emotion, or feeling toward something else or received from someone else in thanks or appreciation.

For some gratitude is a way of life. For others, a journaling practice helps increase a sense of gratitude. Practicing gratitude can help you deal with life's problems by helping you find a sense of meaning, peace, contentment, and purpose, even when dealing with setbacks associated with chronic disease. Gratitude can counter emotional symptoms of depression, help maintain a positive outlook, enhance resiliency, and open the door to creative and effective solutions when problems exist. Researchers studied people with neuromuscular disease, a group of conditions that can cause weakness, muscle paralysis, and breathing, walking, speaking, and swallowing problems. Participants were instructed to keep a 21-day journal recording their sense of well-being and a global assessment of their day. Half the group was also asked to include a record of what they were grateful for each day. The group that focused on gratitude reported a more positive affect, reduced negative affect, and even improved sleep.

Use in Parkinson's

There are many ways that journaling can help people with PD, similar to the way it's been shown to help individuals living with neuromuscular disease:

- *Time to focus:* Organizing thoughts, events, priorities, and expectations helps you focus and reach your goals.
- *Time to yourself:* Think of this time as your quality time—time to think about what is important to you, your wants, desires, successes, disappointments, fears, and struggles
- *Time for self-exploration and introspection:* Journaling brings meaning to the simple and everyday experiences.
- *Emotionally healing:* PD can lead to many ups and downs for you and the whole family. Journaling is one way to help you and your family or loved ones through the bad times and chronicle the good times. It can help you process your emotions and deal with daily stress. For some, journaling can improve mood and stress.
- *Therapeutic:* People who experience emotional or stressful events but do not express, share, or communicate their emotions—otherwise called type D personalities—may be at increased risk for health problems. Journaling is especially helpful for people with chronic conditions or caregivers that tend to hold things in and tend not to discuss their issues, concerns, or emotions.
- *Legacy worthy:* Journaling creates a legacy of your life story and a family keepsake for future generations to enjoy.

Precautions

Journaling may not be for everyone. Talk to your health care provider to see if it is right for you, especially if you suffer from serious depression, anxiety, or other psychiatric conditions, as journaling can bring deep-seated emotions to the surface.

Guidance

Commit 10 to 15 minutes a day or at least a few times a week to journaling. Like any daily task, it is helpful to develop a routine, perhaps journaling the same time every day. Write honestly and be open about your feelings and thoughts. Include something big or small that you are grateful for each day. Decide whether you would like to keep your entries private or use it as an opportunity to open up discussion or dialogue with family, friends, or your clinicians. Record your entries or use a voice-activated software program such as Dragon Speak if you are unable to type.

MUSIC AND ART THERAPY

Description and Mechanism of Action

The physical benefits of music therapy are discussed in Chapter 7 Body Therapy. Music (including dance) and art therapy can be used as a form of creative expression to enhance physical healing, emotional health, and social connection, as well as to connect with personal identity and enhance self-confidence in the setting of disease, change, or conflict and emotional healing. Music and art therapy have been used for stroke recovery, post-traumatic stress disorder (PTSD), emotional disorders, and cognitive disorders such as dementia.

Art therapy is performed individually or in group sessions. According to the American Art Therapy Association (www.arttherapy.org), art therapists complete a master's degree program in which they are trained in the use of visual arts, creative process, human development, and psychological counseling.

Use in Parkinson's

One of the best ways to understand how art therapy can help people with PD is to understand the benefits of art therapy in other neurologic and emotional conditions. Art therapy may help people to:

- Improve upper extremity range of motion, dexterity, and hand-eye coordination
- Experience freedom of movement
- Improve mood, anxiety, stress management through projects focused on expression of mood
- Explore self-expression not limited by disease, physical problems, labels, or other restrictions
- Find creative expression
- Experience a sense of control and achievement
- Reconnect with personal individuality
- Deal therapeutically with fear, grief, uncertainty, or loss that can come with PD-related change

Precautions

There are few precautions for art and music therapy. These therapies often use movement and creative expression as a way to tap into emotions and conflict that is not always obvious. For some, these emotions may cause distress and a counselor can help deal with any difficult symptoms or feelings that arise.

Guidance

You do not have to be a dancer or artist to benefit from these therapies. In fact, this is a great opportunity to learn new cognitive and sensorimotor skill if you have no experience with art or dance. Information on music therapy and certification of therapists is included in the music therapy section of Chapter 7. Art therapists also receive specialized training including bachelor's or master's degrees. The Art Therapy Credentials Board (www.atcb.org) offers certification for qualified therapists and the American Art Therapy Association offers information about the profession and how to find a therapist.

NATURE OR ECOTHERAPY

Description and Mechanism of Action

We've long known that connecting with nature has a powerful influence. Natural spaces stimulate creativity, engagement, and problem solving, yet at the same time add a sense of peacefulness and calm. Nature gives us a respect for our interconnectedness and adds meaning and purpose to life. Hospitals, hospice programs, and healing arts practitioners now intentionally add nature to their décor and environment to enhance personal healing.

Nature therapy is a growing field of professionals in the healing arts that are using the sights, sounds, and touch of nature in their healing programs.

John Muir, a naturalist and nature lover, once wrote,
"In every walk with nature one receives far more than he seeks."

Use in Parkinson's

Exposure to nature can improve emotional health. Exercise and walking is an important focus for PD. Before you head to the gym to get on the treadmill or a stationary bike, consider exercising outdoors. A study comparing the effect of a 30-minute walk on depression showed an improvement in mood in 71%, and improved self-esteem in 90% of participants when walking in a park. Only 45% showed improved mood when walking in an indoor shopping center; 22% felt more depressed and 50% were more tense. Just as the therapeutic relationship affects outcomes of healing therapies, the environment in which a treatment or therapy is performed also influences the results.

Nature is available to everyone at all stages of PD. As little as five minutes a day in a natural setting, whether walking in the park, gardening, or sitting and gazing at the birds, can improve mood, self-esteem, and motivation. Using nature videos, artwork, and exposure to the outdoors, researchers show that recovery from surgery is faster, the length of hospital stays are reduced, and the healing process is enhanced.

Precautions

There are few problems or risks with experiencing the sounds, sights, and smells of nature. However, certain precautions are important to observe before heading outside:

- Pay attention to the weather and your surroundings to ensure safety.
- Drink plenty of water, especially during the hot days of summer, to avoid dehydration.
- Pace yourself if needed, since fatigue can cause falls.

- Be alert to uneven surfaces that challenge walking and balance. Use a walker with a seat for rest and trekking poles or other ambulatory aids, if needed. Avoid carrying items in your hands and use a small backpack instead if balance is a problem.
- Use sunscreen to protect your skin from damaging UV rays.

Guidance

Follow these simple tips to bring the outdoors into your work space, living space, or to create a healing space if recovering from surgery or illness:

- Add colorful flowers and plants, especially during the gray winter months.
- Use the soothing sounds of nature to help you fall asleep or fight stress.
- Fill your walls with artwork that depicts nature scenes and memories.
- Create an outdoor getaway to get lost in nature. It doesn't have to be an elaborate deck or patio. A well-placed chair outside may be all you need.
- Enjoy the benefits of a small fish tank, potted fern, or bird feeder.
- Use stone, wood, and shells as centerpieces or accents in your home rather than commercially bought items.
- Collect items such as rocks or leaves on your nature trips, as a way to bring your experience home and as a reminder.

The next time you are outdoors, think about how the experience changes how you feel. As examples:

- The fresh air sharpens the senses and clears the mind of clutter.
- The experience of watching nature brings marvel and good-natured fun.
- The peaceful calm of a gentle breeze has a stress-dissolving effect.
- The first spring buds elicit a sense of hope and anticipation.
- The reflection of days past and future anticipation radiate from the sunset or sunrise.
- The challenge and sure-footedness of walking is gained from having uneven ground under foot.
- The experience of being outdoors offers a chance to slow down, share your walk, and connect with a loved one.
- The feel of the sun's warmth on your skin or your back can have an energizing or soothing effect.
- The little things like a bird's song or child's laughter are joyful reminders of what's important in life.

Consider these suggestions to increase your time and connection with the outdoors:

- Spend a few minutes every day outside.
- Focus *all* your senses on the marvels of nature. Be sure to take in the many sights, smells, sounds, touch/feelings that come with the experience.

- Marvel in the small and often overlooked. When was the last time you picked up a leaf and truly examined the veins that make up the structure of the leaf or the intricate patterns of color?

SPIRITUAL HEALING AND PRAYER

Description and Mechanism of Action

Faith healing and prayer are examples of spiritual healing. Prayer solicits the power of faith and belief in a higher power that can comfort, guide, and heal.

Prayer is one of the most common and oldest healing rituals. Over 90% of people with serious illness turn to prayer to treat and recover. Prayer is an intensely personal action based on cultural, religious, and spiritual beliefs. Prayer can be directed with a certain outcome in mind or it can be non-directed. Specific types of prayers used to heal include:

- *Intercessory prayer.* Prayer done on behalf of someone else.
- *Petition prayer.* Prayer asking a higher power for something.
- *Centering and contemplative prayer.* Prayer centered on a word, phrase, or idea such as compassion or relief of suffering.
- *Meditation.* A form of prayer used in some religions to promote union with a higher power, deepening awareness and insight into thoughts, ideas, and personal and spiritual growth.

Research does not support the belief that intercessory prayer, or prayer for others, will improve healing. One of the largest and most comprehensive studies to date was designed to evaluate the effect of intercessory prayer for 1,802 patients undergoing open heart surgery in six hospitals. Congregational members prayed for these patients before and after they underwent open heart surgery. Half of the patients were told they were being prayed for and half were informed they may or may not receive prayers. Major complications were identified in 59% that knew they were being prayed for, 51% that were uncertain about whether they were receiving prayers, and 18% that were not informed. Among a few of the reasons why prayer could increase complications: patients end up being less compliant with medical instructions, depending on prayer instead, or directed prayer has the effect of altering people's perceptions of their disease (being a recipient of prayer could lead patients to spend more time thinking about their disease or focusing on the negative consequences of disease).

Intercessory prayer is very different from personal prayer. Personal prayer such as petition, contemplative, or meditative prayer can have healing benefits. Ways in which these practices heal are by:

- Increasing relaxation response, which can have a multitude of health benefits as described in prior chapters of this book
- Increasing one's sense of control
- Eliciting the placebo effect, brought on by power or expectation and belief

- Reinforcing positive feelings over negative feelings, such as compassion, forgiveness, and generosity
- Kindling a sense of hope or possibility
- Increasing focus on others instead of personal symptoms and disease

How you approach treatment and life with a chronic condition is influenced by spiritual experience and practice. A focus on the physical self becomes increasingly important with advancing disease or end of life, but can lead to feelings of loss and grief. Couple this focus on physical wellness with attention to the spiritual self to give a renewed sense of strength and wholeness.

Precautions

Spiritual practices, including meditation and prayer, can add a sense of meaning at times of uncertainty and a feeling of solace to counter pain and disability and acceptance. Spiritual practices bring people together in a supportive way and offer a wellness focus outside of the physical body.

Faith healers use the power of prayer and belief in place of traditional medical care. Faith healers capitalize on the vulnerability, fear, and desperation of people living with chronic illness. There is no evidence to support the benefits of faith healers. Faith healing should not be confused with spiritual healing, which can be an important part of the holistic care of PD.

Guidance

Spiritual practices are best embraced if they are in line with your own spiritual beliefs.

Spirituality is different from religion and will be different for each person. Pastoral care services can be a tremendous benefit and a place to start. These non-denominational services are often available in hospitals, hospices, nursing homes, and home health care institutions or organizations.

SUPPORT AND SUPPORT GROUPS

Description and Mechanism of Action

Support comes in many forms: family, friends, and spiritual or religious groups, to name a few. Support groups are formed when people with similar concerns or problems come together, usually with the goal of offering advice and improving education or the emotional health of participants. Support groups offer an opportunity for people with similar interests or concerns to:

- Obtain information on PD and treatment.
- Gain emotional support, advice, and tips from others.
- Learn from the experience of others.

- Provide others with information and guidance based on experience with disease.
- Develop a sense of community and partnership.
- Learn about and from other professionals in your area.
- Fight loneliness and anxiety.
- Understand that you are not alone.

Use in Parkinson's

An analysis of patients seen at a movement disorders specialty center showed that support groups are helpful. Of patients who returned a survey, 61% attended at least one group. Of these, 49% were very satisfied with the group. Concerns voiced by 15% included the inability of support groups to address their specific needs and concerns when the group did not have the expertise needed (14%). Support groups can be monthly meetings, impromptu lunches, or online chat rooms. The makeup of a support group may be an important factor that influences outcome—that is, when a group's participants are most similar (e.g., same disease stage, age group), they may be more committed to the group and get greater benefit from the group.

Precautions

Not every support group is for every person. The most common reasons people do not attend support groups are as follows:

- People with early disease just coming to terms with diagnosis may feel distressed when attending a support group consisting of people with advanced symptoms and disease.
- Young-onset individuals may feel they do not have a lot in common with older individuals. Online support groups are available for individuals with young-onset PD if there is not a local group in their area.
- The format of a support group may be too formal, relying on educational lectures only, or conversely, the group may lack any formality or structure.
- The group may be focused more on negative issues and less on positive solutions and support.

Guidance

The following tips can help you find the right support group.

- Think about what type of group fits your needs. Are you more comfortable in a large group, small group, one that is focused on education and lectures, or one that is focused on emotional support? Is the age group diverse? Do the members share a common goal or objective such as exercise, deep brain stimulation, caregiving, fundraising, or advocacy?
- Sample a support group(s) to see how it feels and determine if it is the right fit for you.

- Contact your regional PD group or foundation to learn more about groups available in your area. You can also contact one of the many national organizations such as the National Parkinson Foundation (www.parkinson.org), American Parkinson Disease Association (www.apdaparkinson.org), and the Parkinson's Disease Foundation (www.pdf.org) to learn more.

VOLUNTEERISM

Description

Volunteering does more than just make you feel good. Volunteering is actually good for your health. Volunteerism can be divided into two major categories: altruistic (to benefit others) and egocentric (to help oneself). Some important benefits are as follows:

- Older people (age 60 or older) get the most out of volunteering. This includes improved physical function, cognitive function, and life satisfaction. A study of older adults in California showed that people who volunteered lived longer than those who did not.
- Volunteering helps with the isolation, depression, or adjustment to new role definitions that can occur after retirement.
- Volunteering improves self-confidence and provides a sense of purpose.

Use in Parkinson's

Volunteerism can help reduce depression, expand your social network, and enhance self-esteem. Volunteerism offers an opportunity to redefine personal roles through a renewed sense of purpose.

Guidance

Volunteerism poses many mental health benefits that are meaningful and purposeful. Occupational therapy can help you find volunteer opportunities that are meaningful to you. Think about what interests you or what you are passionate about. Is it your children's educational needs, food and shelter for the hungry, a religious activity, environmental or political advocacy, or support for others with PD? There is no shortage of volunteering opportunities. The most important thing is to believe and feel passionate about what you are supporting.

References

Animal Therapy and Service Dogs

Banks, M. R., and W. A. Banks. 2002. "The effects of animal-assisted therapy on loneliness in an elderly population in long-term care facilities." *The Journals of Gerontology: Series A Biological Sciences and Medical Sciences* 57: M428–32.

Fine, H. A., ed. 2010. "Handbook on animal-assisted therapy: Theoretical foundations and guidelines for practice." San Diego, CA: Academic Press.

Journaling and Gratitude

Emmons, R. A. 2008. "Gratitude, subjective well-being, and the brain." In *The Science of Subjective Well-Being*, edited by M. Eid and R. Larsen. New York, NY: Guilford Press.

Emmons, R., and M. E. McCullough. 2003. "Counting blessings versus burdens: An experimental investigation of gratitude and subjective well-being in daily life." *Journal of Personality and Social Psychology* 84: 377.

Music and Art Therapy

Slayton, S., et al. 2010. "Outcomes studies of the efficacy of art therapy: A review of findings." *Art Therapy: Journal of the American Art Therapy Association* 27: 108–18.

Nature or Ecotherapy

Pryor, A., et al. 2006. "Health and well-being naturally: 'Contact with nature' in health promotion for targeted individuals, communities, and populations." *Health Promotion Journal of Australia* 17: 114–23.

Study published by Mind, www.org.uk

Spiritual Healing and Prayer

Bay, P. S. 2008. "The effect of pastoral care services on anxiety, depression, hope, religious coping, and religious problem-solving styles: A randomized controlled study." *Journal of Religion and Health* 47: 57–69.

Benson, H., et al. 2006. "Study of the therapeutic effects of intercessory prayer (STEP) in cardiac bypass patients: A multicenter randomized trial of uncertainty and certainty of receiving intercessory prayer." *American Heart Journal* 151: 934–42.

Support and Support Groups

Dorsey, E. R., et al. 2010. "A U.S. survey of patients with Parkinson's disease: Satisfaction with medical care and support groups." *Movement Disorders* 25: 2128–35.

Lieberman, M. A., et al. 2005. "The impact of group composition on Internet support groups: Homogeneous versus heterogeneous Parkinson's groups." *Group Dynamics: Theory, Research, and Practice* 2005: 239–50.

Volunteerism

Black, W., and R. Living. 2004. "Volunteerism as an occupation and its relationship to health and wellbeing." *British Journal of Occupational Therapy* 67: 526–32.

Lum, T. Y., and E. Lightfoot 2005. "The effects of volunteering on the physical and mental health of older people." *Research on Aging* 27: 31–35.

Oman, D., et al. 1999. "Volunteerism and mortality among the community-dwelling elderly." *Journal of Health Psychology* 4: 301–16.

CHAPTER 11

Whole System Approaches

By now, I hope you understand that integrative medicine is not a collection of treatments, healing arts, or practitioners but a philosophy of care that embraces the scientific benefits of traditional medicine with personal healing based on balance, intention, empowerment, and emotional and spiritual healing. The idea that health is enhanced when cellular physiology, organ system control, and physical and emotional states are in balance with the needs of your body, mind, and spiritual is not new. In fact, as new as integrative medicine appears, it is as old as the earliest teachings of health and disease.

The evolution and existence of modern-day Western medicine is shaped in part by discoveries beginning in the 19th century: the understanding that pathogens such as bacteria cause disease, the discovery of antibiotics, and advances in surgery necessitated by injuries sustained in military battles. What followed these discoveries was a directed approach away from the individual as a whole and toward the identification and treatment of disease by isolating symptoms and cellular causes. This approach has led to the discovery of even greater medical and surgical therapies. The incredible breakthroughs that are a product of Westernized medicines should not be shunned, just as the thoughtful embrace of alternative medicines should not be criticized.

What is emerging is a "new" version of modern-day medicine, one in which these theories, ideas, and concepts could and should be integrated with age-old systems embracing interconnectedness, wholeness, and emotional well-being. In effect, traditional medicine offers a focus on treatment (akin to looking into a microscope) that hones in on the damage, deficits, and abnormal genetic, cellular, and chemical processes associated with disease, while integrative approaches expand and broaden the lens to focus more broadly on the emotional well-being, personal healing, and supportive and spiritual health of the person as a whole.

One of the key differences between traditional medicine and whole systems approaches is the inclusion of the whole body as a system and focus of health and the reliance on emotional, social, cultural, spiritual, and environment influences. In this chapter, we review a few commonly practiced whole systems approaches that have been in existence over the millennia and are now being applied to the "new" idea of integrative medicine. Originating in ancient times, these systems describe health and disease without the understanding of physiology, pathology, genetics, and environmental science as known today. These systems do, however, provide a bridging philosophy that reinforces the strong interconnection of these individual approaches.

AYURVEDIC MEDICINE

Description and Mechanism of Action

Over 2,000 years old, Ayurvedic medicine is one of the oldest systems of medicine. Ayurveda, or *life knowledge*, is Sanskrit for *ayur* (life) and *veda* (science or knowledge). Like other ancient medical systems, Ayurveda supports the idea that health is influenced by the interconnectedness of people, the environment or larger world, and an individual's life forces and body constitution. Ayurveda is often referred to as life wisdom, since it includes guidance on daily habits that change with seasonal change, as well as compassionate and ethical living practices. In some situations health or illness is related to constant changes and interactions between these forces; in other situations, a person's constitution (which does not change) plays a primary role in health and disease. Two unique features of Ayurvedic medicine are the concepts of *prana* and *dosha*:

- *Prana* is the life force that supports the body and is vital to life. This life force is nourished by the lungs and intestines, which absorb oxygen and food or life. For this reason, many Ayurvedic therapies focus on working with the breath and diet.

- *Dosha* refers to a person's unique life force or energy. Illness can occur if a person's dosha is in overabundance or in deficit. Each person has a unique balance of three doshas that define their temperament or constitution: *vata, pitta,* and *kapha*. This balance represents the person's unique state in the setting of health.

- *Vata* or energy of movement includes the energy of breathing and the heart. People with this pattern are often thin and energetic, alert, flexible, and creative. When *vata* is out of balance this pattern can revert to anxiety, muscle twitches, and other neurologic problems.

- *Pitta* or energy of action includes the energy of digestion and hormones. People with this pattern are typically more intense in nature and goal and action oriented. When *pitta* is out of balance, agitation or anger can result as well as disease associated with inflammation, ulcers, and fever.

- *Kapha* or the energy of strength and growth includes the energy of immunity and growth. People with this pattern have a muscular body habitus and possess strength and endurance. When *kapha* is out of balance, fatigue or lethargy can occur as well as diseases of congestion.

Initial treatment will often focus on rebalancing the doshas, eliminating toxins, improving digestion, and addressing lifestyle habits including diet, activity, levels of stress, relationships, and coping strategies. Specific treatments often include herbal therapies, massage, dosha-specific diets, fasting and purging, yoga, meditation, and counseling. Balance is emphasized, as is moderation of activities such as diet, sleep, and sex.

Use in Parkinson's

Ayurvedic approaches toward Parkinson's disease (PD) in the United States tend to fall into the categories of yoga, diet, elimination, and herbal therapies.

Three Ayurvedic plant-based compounds commonly used to treat PD are mucuna pruriens (cowhage seeds), brahmi (Bacopa), and curcumin (turmeric).

- Mucuna pruriens is the most common herbal preparation used in PD, chosen as a natural source of levodopa. In a placebo-controlled trial, mucuna pruriens exhibited a more rapid onset to peak dose and longer duration of "on" time without an increase in dyskinesia, suggesting that there are additional benefits beyond levodopa obtained when taking this herbal medicine.

- Brahmi *(Bacopa monniera)* is thought to improve brain circulation, mood, and cognitive function. For this reason, it is a popular Ayurvedic herb for use with neurologic conditions including PD. There are no studies, however, to support the use of this herb for PD.

- Curcumin is the active component in turmeric, a common spice used in Indian curry dishes. Curcumin is a polyphenol, which is a chemical class of medicines that can penetrate the blood-brain barrier and gain access to brain cells. Research suggests that curcumin has strong anti-inflammatory and antioxidant properties and can rescue proteins from clumping or aggregating in cells, making curcumin worth further study for neurodegenerative diseases, including PD and Alzheimer's disease. Studies to date are on animals and the evidence or dose for use in people is not yet available.

Rasayana, or the science of rejuvenation, refers to an Ayurvedic approach focused on the prevention and treatment of disease and slowing of the aging process. As such, it is an Ayurvedic branch used to treat age-related neurodegenerative diseases such as Alzheimer's disease and PD. Herbal compounds used for this purpose are classified as rejuvenators, many of which exhibit strong antioxidant properties, supporting the need for further study of potential benefits.

Precautions

There is no certain evidence that Ayurvedic medicine as a whole is beneficial to PD symptoms or quality of life. However, certain Ayurvedic philosophies and practices could be of benefit if approached in a thoughtful way. For instance, a personalized and holistic approach to care that includes a focus on balance and moderation, positive lifestyle change, and practices to strengthen mind and body are proven effective. Certain Ayurvedic practices such as fasting and oral (vomiting) or colon (laxatives) purging are risky and should not be performed. Tremor associated with hypoglycemia, light-headedness and low blood pressure, loss of energy or strength, decline in mood, weight loss, or reduced activity and exercise performance could result.

Ayurvedic diets are often prescribed based on an individual's unique doshas. Caution is advised, especially if one plans to adopt dietary recommendations without first reviewing them with your health care provider.

Herbal preparations are an important part of Ayurvedic medicine. Mucuna pruriens, a natural source of levodopa, and other herbal compounds are used for the treatment of PD. Remember that clinical studies are (ideally) performed with the highest-grade herbal compounds, ensuring purity and potency. This is not the case with herbal products marketed to consumers. A team of researchers from Boston University School of Medicine tested Ayurvedic herbal supplements produced in India and the United States and marketed in the States or via the Internet. Of the products tested, 21% contained lead, mercury, or arsenic that exceeded acceptable standards. The Centers for Disease Control and Prevention reported 12 cases of lead poisoning associated with Ayurvedic products between 2000 and 2003.

Guidance

Remember that herbal therapies are and should be thought of as medicines and placed in the same category as prescription medicines. Involve your health care provider in any decision to use Ayurvedic herbal medicines. Consider taking prescription-form levodopa rather than mucuna pruriens to ensure you are receiving a safe product with predictable and stable strength across doses. Discuss your concerns about safety with your doctor and avoid treatments that are not tested for safety in standardized laboratories. Begin first by focusing on Ayurvedic principles and therapies with proven benefit and low risk, such as the principles of balance and moderation. Consider beginning with yoga, mind-body therapies, and sound dietary changes instead of herbal treatments. Seek Ayurvedic specialists who are adequately trained. Unfortunately, there are many different training programs, so experience and expertise will vary considerable. Some Ayurvedic specialists are doctors, nutritionists, or nurses with medical training who received additional training in medicine and this method. As always, be sure that you review any changes with your health care provider.

HOMEOPATHY

Description and Mechanism of Action

Unlike other whole system approaches with Eastern origins described in this section, homeopathy originated in Western Europe. Christian Friedrich Samuel Hahnemann received his medical degree in 1779 but soon left medicine as he thought it did just as much harm as good. During his research as a writer and translator he discovered a claim that the astringent properties of cinchona, the bark of a Peruvian tree, could treat malaria. He also understood that other tonics with astringent properties did not treat malaria. His research led him to conduct his own experiments. When he ingested cinchona, he experienced malaria-like symptoms of fever, sweating, fatigue. This experience led to the theory that a treatment that can produce symptoms similar to the disease could be used to heal the disease. This is known as "like cures like." One problem, however, is that many of these compounds are toxic. He solved this dilemma by diluting treatments to concentrations that would not have these toxic effects as they contain an unmeasurable trace of the original compound. What is left behind is a chemical or functional memory of the molecular structure of the original compound.

In summary, homeopathy is based on these three principles:

1. *Like treats like:* What causes symptoms can treat symptoms.
2. *Individualization of treatment:* Treatment is tailored to the physical, emotional, and personal traits of the individual.
3. *Minimum dose:* Aggressive dilution and vigorous shaking with each dilution is an important part of a solution's effectiveness.

The acceptance of homeopathy as a legitimate science and/or treatment is controversial. An important part of the placebo effect is the involvement of the practitioner's belief and the patient's expectation of a treatment. The same can be stated for homeopathic therapy, which is a similar albeit different process. An article in *Recent Advances in Computer Science* described it this way: "In homeopathy attention falls on the remedy that in undiluted state has the capacity of inducing the same effects as the pathogenic factor, thus determining its replacement in the newly created psychological space of the bad disturbing agent by the good harmless remedy, which does not fight against it, but only replaces it in its effects, by preventing it to draw attention and produce psychological effects." Homeopathic practitioners argue that homeopathy is indeed both grounded in solid scientific principles and a legitimate medical therapy. Yet there are limited controlled studies to support these claims, and a review of the studies performed showed that less positive results were found in studies when controlled research methods were used.

Use in Parkinson's

Homeopathy is a common alternative therapy used by people with PD. Individual reports or observations of benefit are reported on the Internet, but no studies have been performed. Therefore, there is no evidence to support the use of this therapy.

Precautions

As noted, there is no evidence to support the use of homeopathic preparations for PD. It is important to note that the Food and Drug Administration (FDA) does not limit the amount of alcohol allowed in these preparations (less than 10% is the limit for other products and medicines) and alcohol could account for acute affects. Do not use if you have concerns for or a history of alcohol abuse.

Guidelines

Understand first that there is no evidence to support use of these products for PD. Talk to your health care provider before starting a homeopathic therapy.

TRADITIONAL CHINESE MEDICINE

Description and Mechanism of Action

Traditional Chinese medicine (TCM) dates back to Taoism over 2,500 years ago and is based on the philosophy that everything is interrelated. Traditional definitions and concepts of Chinese medicine are difficult to translate into modern-day language and perhaps should not be interpreted. Instead, a general understanding of the concepts could prove valuable as a foundation for understanding the importance of health from the point of view of the body and spirit as a whole. The following are important TCM concepts:

Wholeness: Organs are definite structures, but their function and actions cannot be separated from one another. The health of one organ will affect other organs. Healing occurs when treating the person not the disease. Organs cannot be separated nor can the mind be separated from the body. Together they form an energy system that must exist in balance within the body but also in union with the environment and world.

Yin and Yang: These opposite but complementary states exist together as a balance. This balance is in constant flux. Nothing is all yin or all yang and the two can change into one another. Qualities attributed to yin include female, earth, cold, winter, night, chronicity, and moisture. Qualities attributed to yang include male, celestial, warmth, summer, day, acuteness, and dryness.

Vital Substances: These substances make up and nourish the body and mind. These substances are *Qi* (energy or life force, blood, other body fluids), Jing (vital life force or constitution), and Shen (mind or spirit).

Internal Organs: Organs are categorized into five elements present in the world around us: wood, fire, earth, metal, and water. Organs are also divided into solid and hollow organs, yin and yang organs. Different organs play a role in or store vital substances.

Meridians: Organs and vital substances are connected by energy channels that travel throughout the body called meridians. Flow and balance of energy along these meridians is a basis for the practice of acupuncture.

Chinese medicine uses four techniques to examine a patient:

1. *Pulse:* strength, regularity, rhythm
2. *Inspection:* skin, facial inspection, tongue, body habitus, body language, and behavior
3. *Listen:* speech volume and quality, breathing and coughing
4. *Inquire:* review of a person's medical history and experience

Taken together, TCM places great emphasis on what can be learned by the appearance and presence of the person (physically and emotionally), the power of communication and personal experience, the concept of balance (physically, emotionally, and spiritually), and finally the idea that these subtle findings are interrelated, just as the body as a whole is dependent on the health of all organ systems.

Use in Parkinson's

The majority of studies evaluating the effect of TCM on PD symptoms has focused on two specific treatment modalities: acupuncture (Chapter 9) and tai chi (Chapter 7). Other studies evaluate the specific effects of herbal preparations. The very essence of TCM, however, is not in the use of structured therapies but in the tailoring of therapies based on the emotional, physical, and spiritual state of the person. This holistic and individualized approach that treats the person means that treatment will be very different from one person to the next even when treating the same disease or symptoms.

Ancient medical texts describe conditions with "trembling of the hands" in aging. Theory states that reduced yin in the kidney and liver is related to symptoms of aging and reduced strength in the spleen and stomach is associated with PD. Treatments and herbal drugs have therefore been used in the treatment of

PD under the general guideline of "strengthening the spleen and regulating the stomach."

One study examined the effect of a 24-week course of a Chinese herbal medicine formula on motor and non-motor symptoms, and on complications of conventional therapy in PD, using an add-on design. Like many TCM herbal preparations, this treatment is complex, composed of 11 herbs traditionally used to treat symptoms similar to parkinsonism. Ability to communicate and measures of the Unified PD Rating Scale part 4 (measuring symptoms such as nausea, GI distress, and hypotension) showed improvement compared to placebo.

Precautions

Similar to other supplements, Chinese herbs are not regulated as medicines. This means that there are herbal preparations obtained from China that may not meet safety standards for strength and purity. Some herbal preparations sold in the United States were found to be contaminated by heavy metals. Others were found to be adulterated with other medicines such as the blood thinner warfarin, the pain medicine ibuprofen, the energy/appetite suppressant ephedra, or the chemical ephedrine. As noted in the aforementioned research study, herbal preparations often have 10 to 30 different chemicals present in one treatment, making the combined effect on health unknown and very difficult to study. In addition, many treatments are proprietary blends, meaning the true combination and quantities of herbs or chemicals are protected and not available.

Guidance

Remember that herbal therapies are and should be thought of as medicines and should be placed in the same risk category as prescription medicines. Involve your health care provider in any decision to use TCM medicines. Overall lack of direct information on safety, drug interactions, and benefits means herbal therapies have high risk. Discuss your concerns about safety with your doctor and avoid treatments that are not tested for safety in standardized laboratories. Consider focusing on TCM-based mind-body or energy therapies instead of herbal treatments. Seek TCM specialists who are adequately trained. For example, consider acupuncturists who are health care providers, such as medical doctors, and have obtained additional training in acupuncture medicine (usually 500 or more hours) or individuals who have undergone specific training. The National Certification Commission for Acupuncture and Oriental Medicine (www.nccaom.org) offers specific competency criteria for members or diplomats. There is not a specific doctoral degree as multiple doctoral programs exist in the United States. Each program is likely to have a different emphasis and training experience. Examples include doctor of oriental medicine (OMD and DOM), doctor of acupuncture and oriental medicine (DAOM). The Council of Colleges of Acupuncture and Oriental Medicine (www.ccaom.org) is an accreditation organization to ensure U.S. schools offer quality education and training.

INTERVIEW WITH THE EXPERT: ACUPUNCTURE

A MOVEMENT DISORDERS NEUROLOGIST SHARES HIS JOURNEY FROM NEUROLOGY TO ACUPUNCTURE

How did you get started in your work with acupuncture?

During my final year of high school, I took a course in mindfulness meditation at the University of Massachusetts Medical Center with Jon Kabat-Zinn and Saki Santorelli. Over time, my interests in integrative medicine expanded, and as I entered medical school, I began to learn more about acupuncture. In particular, I became especially interested after professors told me about bringing their pets for acupuncture. A dog certainly was not expecting any good to come from being brought to a doctor who stuck needles into him. If the dog felt pain relief, I thought that there must be something happening beyond a placebo response. I then began to spend time shadowing doctors who utilized acupuncture as part of their medical practices. I became convinced that this was a treatment modality that I wanted to be able to offer my patients.

Following my neurology residency, I did a fellowship in PD and other movement disorders. During this year I also studied Kiiko Matsumoto's Japanese style of acupuncture in the "Structural Acupuncture for Physicians" course at Harvard Medical School. Since completing my fellowship in 2006, I have been practicing both acupuncture and movement disorders neurology. I find that my patients appreciate and benefit from this broader perspective.

How can this therapy potentially help people with Parkinson's?

My experience has been that acupuncture is most helpful in dealing with the non-motor symptoms of PD. It appears to be helpful in improving sleep quality, increasing energy, decreasing anxiety, and dealing with pain. These are symptoms that are often difficult to treat with pharmaceutical medications.

(continued)

INTERVIEW WITH THE EXPERT (continued)

What would a participant expect during sessions?

I practice a Japanese style of acupuncture, which emphasizes the use of palpation to determine which points will be needled to help restore balance. I ask that my patients dress in comfortable, loose clothing to allow me to access the acupuncture points, most of which are on the arms, hands, legs, feet, and back. Patients may feel a little pinprick or nothing but pressure with needle insertion. Afterward, they will sometimes feel a sensation of deep warmth, or an aching, such as that experienced with a deep muscle massage, arising and spreading from the acupuncture point. This sensation is called *de-qi*, or "the calling of the energy." The needles are then left in place for 10 to 15 minutes and followed by one or two additional sets of needles. The entire session lasts from 60 to 90 minutes. Most of my patients find the experience of an acupuncture session to be very relaxing.

In the United States, most acupuncturists practice a style of acupuncture derived from TCM. These acupuncture treatments differ in some ways, but the overall experience is similar.

How is acupuncture different from other healing therapies?

Acupuncture differs from most Western healing modalities in its emphasis on restoring balance to the person as a whole. Individual symptoms are taken in the context of many factors, including aggravating and alleviating influences, a person's likes and dislikes, and general disposition. The acupuncturist attempts to identify and to remove blockages in the proper flow of energy, "*qi*," throughout the body. In so doing, the body is supported and allowed to better perform its ongoing job of maintaining its health. Acupuncture works best when it is thought of as one tool among many for improving health, rather than an external "fix" or cure. Exercise, social interaction, good nutrition, and medications remain crucial elements of the larger treatment plan.

How do you find a practitioner?

Primary care physicians and/or neurologists may know of a good acupuncturist that their patients have used. Additionally, organizations such as the American Academy of Medical Acupuncture (www .medicalacupuncture.org) and the National Certification Commission

(continued)

INTERVIEW WITH THE EXPERT (*continued*)

for Acupuncture and Oriental Medicine (www.nccaom.org) maintain databases of certified practitioners on their websites that are searchable by location.

What special certification or training should a practitioner have?

An MD who practices acupuncture should have completed an acupuncture training program of at least 300 hours combining coursework and practical bedside learning. Other acupuncturists should have completed a four-year program in Oriental Medicine from a school accredited by the Accreditation Commission for Acupuncture and Oriental Medicine (www.acaom.org). Additionally, they should have state licensure to practice acupuncture.

Adam Simmons, MD, DABIHM

Dr. Simmons is a movement disorders neurologist and the director of the Parkinson's Disease Center at the Hospital for Special Care in New Britain, Connecticut.

References

Ayurvedic Medicine

Katzenschlager, R., et al. 2004. "Mucuna pruriens in Parkinson's disease: A double-blind clinical and pharmacological study." *Journal of Neurology, Neurosurgery, and Psychiatry* 75: 1672–77.

Mythri, R. B., and N. M. Bharath. 2012. "Curcumin: A potential neuroprotective agent in Parkinson's disease." *Current Pharmaceutical Design* 18: 91–99.

Saper, R. B., et al. 2004. "Heavy metal content of Ayurvedic herbal medicine products." *Journal of the American Medical Association* 292: 2868–73.

———. 2008. "Lead, mercury, and arsenic in U.S. and Indian-manufactured Ayurvedic medicines sold over the Internet." *Journal of the American Medical Association* 300: 915–23.

Homeopathy

Filipov, U. S. 2013. "Aspects involved in the cognitive mechanism of the placebo effect versus homeopathy." *Recent Advances in Computer Science.* http://www.wseas.us/e-library/conferences/2013/Rhodes/COMPUTE/COMPUTE-45.pdf

Klaus, L., et al. 1999. "Impact of study quality on outcome in placebo-controlled trials of homeopathy." *Journal of Clinical Epidemiology* 52: 631–36.

Mastrangelo, D. 2007. "Hormesis, epitaxy, the structure of liquid water, and the science of homeopathy." *Medical Science Monitor* 13: S R1–8.

Pecci, C., et al. 2010. "Use of complementary and alternative therapies in outpatients with Parkinson's disease in Argentina." *Movement Disorders* 25: 2094–98.

Traditional Chinese Medicine

Kum, W. F., et al. 2011. "Treatment of idiopathic Parkinson's disease with traditional Chinese herbal medicine: A randomized placebo-controlled pilot clinical study." *Evidence-Based Complementary and Alternative Medicine*: 724353.

Li, A., D. Zhao, and E. Bezard. 2006. "Traditional Chinese medicine for Parkinson's disease: A review of Chinese literature." *Behavioral Pharmacology* 17: 403–10.

Zheng, G. Q. 2009. "Therapeutic history of Parkinson's disease in Chinese medical treatises." *Journal of Alternative and Complementary Medicine* 15: 1223–30.

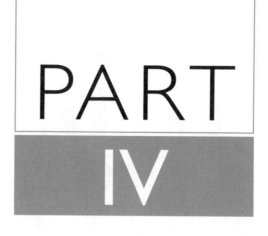

PART

IV

Symptom Relief

So far we have reviewed some of the more common therapies and the rationale for their use in Parkinson's disease (PD). In this section, attention is focused on specific symptoms and their treatments.

Traditional therapies are included since true integration often requires a holistic approach that combines medical and surgical therapies with other treatments you have learned about in this book. In most cases, therapies listed are already explained in detail in earlier chapters. Those that have not are described further in this section. Not all therapies are listed for each symptom. Some therapies lack the evidence to verify safety and are therefore not included here. The following symptoms will be reviewed:

- *Motor Symptoms:* These symptoms include the common problems of tremor, rigidity, bradykinesia, walking, speech, and balance problems.

- *Non-Motor Symptoms:* These important problems are often undiagnosed and untreated. The main categories of non-motor symptoms include cognitive and behavioral symptoms, sleep problems, pain, and sensory and autonomic dysfunction.

CHAPTER

12

Therapies for Motor Symptoms

Motor symptoms of Parkinson's disease (PD) include tremor, rigidity, and brady-kinesia. Medications that enhance the dopamine system are effective for these early symptoms and will be reviewed briefly as they are an important part of your therapy. Walking, balance, speech, and swallowing problems emerge as the disease progress. As PD advances, these symptoms do not respond to standard dopamine medicines and greater emphasis is placed on non-medical therapies. This chapter reviews both traditional and integrative therapies to help you individualize your care.

BRADYKINESIA AND RIGIDITY

Overview

Bradykinesia and rigidity are two of the cardinal symptoms of PD. Combined, these problems can cause difficulty with handwriting and the dexterity of finger movements and spontaneous facial expression (masked face) and can cause slowed movement and decreased arm swing.

Traditional Therapies

Dopaminergic medicines are the most effective treatment for these symptoms, since the symptoms progress as dopaminergic nerve cells degenerate. As the disease progresses, deep brain stimulation (DBS) can help effectively in increasing medicine "on" time and reducing medicine "off" time. Physical therapy can be especially helpful in improving motor symptoms at each disease stage. A review of dopaminergic medicines is included in Chapter 2. These medicines are also summarized in the following table.

EARLY DISEASE*	MID-STAGE DISEASE**	LATE DISEASE***
MAO-B Inhibitors	MAO-B Inhibitors	MAO-B Inhibitors
Dopamine Agonists	Dopamine Agonists	
Carbidopa/Levodopa	Carbidopa/Levodopa	Carbidopa/Levodopa
	COMT Inhibitors	COMT Inhibitors
	Amantadine	
	Deep Brain Stimulation	

*In early disease, multiple medicines can be used. It is sometimes helpful to follow a levodopa-sparing strategy using MAO-B inhibitors or agonists first and adding levodopa medicines when symptoms progress. This strategy levodopa is added in combination, when needed, often at a lower dose. Lower-dose levodopa can reduce or delay the development of dyskinesia. Since levodopa is the most effective medicine for movement, this strategy supports earlier use with lowest risk.

There is a common misconception that levodopa benefit wears off in 5 years and/or levodopa is toxic to nerve cells. Fortunately neither are true, further supporting earlier use of this medicine.

**In mid-stage disease, treatment is focused on increasing on time, reducing off time, and minimizing or reducing medicine-induced dyskinesia and side effects. COMT inhibitors such as entacapone (Comtan®, Stalevo®) can help increase the duration of the levodopa effect. Amantadine can reduce dyskinesia. Duopa carbidopa/levodopa delivered via an intestinal pump is a newly approved treatment helpful for motor fluctuations or dyskinesia. Deep brain stimulation can improve on time, tremor, and dyskinesia.

***In late disease stage, all medicines and surgery can be helpful. However, side effects become a significant problem as medicine dose is increased. This is especially a concern if cognitive problems, hallucinations, or hyper-somnolence are noted. Certain symptoms such as postural instability, freezing of gait, speech and swallowing problems become less responsive to medicine and medicine increase may not be appropriate. The medicines listed in the Late Disease column have a lower risk of these potentially harmful side effects.

Integrative Therapies

LIFESTYLE	SUPPLEMENTS	BODY	MIND-BODY	ENERGY	OTHER
Foods*	Mucuna Pruriens***	Yoga	Meditation		Support Group
Exercise**	Citicholine	Tai Chi	Guided Imagery		
	Glutathione	Dance and Music			
	Marijuana	Massage****			

(*continued*)

Integrative Therapies (*continued*)

*Foods associated with reduced risk of PD have not been proven to reduce symptoms once present or progression. Diets such as the Mediterranean diet, a vegetarian diet, and foods such as green tea, coffee, peppers, and berries may reduce PD risk.

**Exercise can help in many ways. To date, high-intensity physical activities, weight training, yoga, tai chi, dance, and music therapy are noted to improve symptoms.

***Mucuna pruriens contains levodopa. Concerns include supplement purity and problems with consistent dosing from one dose to the other.

****Massage (also chiropractic and acupuncture) should not be performed near the area of the battery (usually under the collarbone), neck, and head in people who have deep brain stimulation (DBS) implants.

DYSKINESIA

Overview

Dyskinesia is uncontrollable or involuntary movement caused by dopaminergic medicines, most notably levodopa. Dyskinesia can improve by reducing dopaminergic medicines, yet this strategy alone is often accompanied by increased motor off time.

Traditional Therapies

Carbidopa/levodopa is often reduced or used in smaller, more frequent doses to minimize dyskinesia noted at peak dose (usually about one hour post-levodopa dose). Other medications such as MAO-B inhibitors, dopamine agonists, or COMT inhibitors can improve on time, thus allowing a reduction in levodopa total daily dose. Amantadine is unique since this medicine can both improve motor symptoms and, in some patients, reduce dyskinesia. Rytary is a new form of extended release carbidopa/levodopa that can improve motor on time and dyskinesia. Duopa is a gel preparation of levodopa infused via pump into the intestines for treatment of motor fluctuations and dyskinesia. DBS is also effective when motor fluctuations and/or dyskinesia are experienced.

Integrative Therapies

LIFESTYLE	SUPPLEMENTS	BODY	MIND-BODY	ENERGY	OTHER
Foods	Mucuna Pruriens**	Yoga	Meditation		Support Group
Exercise*	Citicholine	Tai Chi	Music Therapy		
	Glutathione	Dance and Music			
	Naltrexone	Massage***			

(continued)

Integrative Therapies (*continued*)

*Exercise can help in many ways. To date, high-intensity activities, weight training, yoga, tai chi, dance, and music therapy are noted to improve symptoms.

**Mucuna pruriens contains levodopa. Concerns include supplement purity and problems with consistent dosing from one dose to the other.

***Massage (also chiropractic and acupuncture) should not be performed near the area of the battery (usually under the collarbone), neck, and head in people who have DBS implants.

TREMOR

Overview

Tremor can accompany rigidity and bradykinesia but is not present in every individual. Tremor can sometimes be difficult to treat, responding less to dopaminergic medicines than bradykinesia or rigidity. Tremor is also very sensitive to stress. Emotional and physical stress, and the stress of another medical disease, can quickly and significantly increase tremor. For this reason, mind-body and stress management techniques can play a particular role in treating this problem.

Traditional Therapies

Dopaminergic and anticholinergic medicines (see Chapter 2) are the most effective medical treatment for these symptoms. Anticholinergic agents are medicines that block the neurotransmitter acetylcholine and are an additional class of medicines that can be used especially in younger patients. However, side effects often limit anticholinergic use. These side effects include:

- Cognitive: memory problems, confusion, hallucinations
- Dryness: eyes and mouth
- Constipation
- Bladder emptying
- Blurry vision
- Low blood pressure, causing dizziness

Occupational therapy is often overlooked but can be very effective in helping with activities and chores (such as eating, typing, writing, or dressing) that are otherwise compromised by tremor.

Integrative Therapies

LIFESTYLE	SUPPLEMENTS	BODY	MIND-BODY	ENERGY	OTHER
Foods	Mucuna Pruriens**	Yoga	Meditation	Reiki	Support Group
Exercise*	Citicholine	Tai Chi	Guided Imagery	Acupuncture	

(*continued*)

Integrative Therapies (*continued*)

LIFESTYLE	SUPPLEMENTS	BODY	MIND-BODY	ENERGY	OTHER
	Glutathione	Dance and Music	Hypnosis		
		Massage***			

*Exercise can help in many ways. Weight training, yoga, tai chi, dance, and music therapy are noted to improve symptoms. High-intensity exercise appears to be especially helpful for tremor.

**Mucuna pruriens contains levodopa. Concerns include supplement purity and problems with consistent dosing from one dose to the other.

***Massage (also chiropractic and acupuncture) should not be performed near the area of the battery (usually under the collarbone), neck, and head in people who have DBS implants.

WALKING, BALANCE, AND FREEZING OF GAIT

Overview

Walking, balance, and freezing of gait are more problematic in the late disease stage. Although initially improved with medicine, these symptoms progress and become refractory or unresponsive to dopaminergic medicines.

Traditional Therapies

In late stage, these symptoms do not respond to dopaminergic medicine. Care must be taken to avoid medicine increase as this strategy will only increase side effects. Side effects that cause problems especially in later stages are confusion, hallucinations, impulse control, sedation, and light-headedness. Physical and occupational therapy are very important at this stage, with the goal of improving symptoms, adjusting and adapting to changes, and prescribing ambulatory aids for safety.

Integrative Therapies

LIFESTYLE	SUPPLEMENTS	BODY	MIND-BODY	ENERGY	OTHER
Foods	Vitamin D	Yoga	Meditation	Whole Body Vibration	Support Group
Exercise*	Vitamin B12	Tai Chi	Imagery		Nature Therapy
		Dance and Music			Pet Therapy
		Massage			
		Alexander Technique®			

*Community-based exercise can help in many ways. Dance, music therapy, yoga, and tai chi have been shown to improve balance in clinical research.

CHAPTER

13

Therapies for Non-Motor Symptoms

Non-motor symptoms can be significant. Studies show these symptoms can contribute to quality of life as much or sometimes even more than motor symptoms. This finding further supports the need for a holistic and individualized care approach that extends beyond the motor symptoms of Parkinson's disease (PD). Integrative therapies are especially effective when coupled with traditional therapies for many of these non-motor problems. The more common non-motor symptoms include cognitive and behavioral symptoms, sleep problems, pain, and sensory and autonomic dysfunction. Causes of non-motor symptoms are diverse and include:

- Changes in brain physiology and chemistry
- Medication-induced side effects (as outlined in Chapter 2)
- Emotional reaction to living with a chronic disease
- Lifestyle changes associated with PD (such as a more sedentary lifestyle).

ANXIETY

Overview

Anxiety can occur as a symptom of the disease, reaction to loss of abilities, or fear of change. Anxiety could be generalized, experienced during specific times such as during gait freezing, or noted as a non-motor fluctuation (often experienced at end of dose) and as an abrupt panic attack. Anxiety often occurs with depression. Anxiety can cause many symptoms including a sense of nervousness or doom, restlessness, insomnia, abdominal pain and diarrhea, shortness of breath, and rapid heart rate. Anxiety will also worsen motor symptoms especially tremor, rigidity, dystonia, dyskinesia, and freezing of gait.

Anxiety is associated with an increase in the stress response, essentially boosting the sympathetic nervous system and decreasing the parasympathetic nervous system and response. Many treatments are aimed at resetting the balance by reducing the sympathetic nervous system and enhancing the parasympathetic nervous system.

Traditional Therapies

These therapies usually include a combination of counseling (talk therapy) and medication. Cognitive behavioral therapy is described in a subsequent section on "depression" later in this chapter. Common medical therapies include benzodiazepines and selective serotonin reuptake inhibitors (SSRIs).

Integrative Therapies

LIFESTYLE	SUPPLEMENTS	BODY	MIND-BODY	ENERGY	OTHER
Foods	Tryptophan	Yoga	Breathwork	Reiki	Support Group
Exercise*	Herbs: Lavender, Lemon Balm, and Valerian Root	Tai Chi	Meditation	Acupuncture	Pet Therapy
	St. John's Wort	Dance and Music	Guided Imagery	Aromatherapy	Journaling
	GABA	Massage	Biofeedback		Music and Art Therapy
					Nature Therapy

*Exercise can help in many ways. High-intensity exercise is especially helpful when depression is also present. Tai chi, dance. and yoga are exercises that place particular emphasis on the relaxation response.

APATHY

Overview

Apathy is a loss of motivation to engage in activities and complete tasks. Apathy is a symptom of the disease or can occur with or without depression or dementia.

Apathy can sometimes be misinterpreted as disinterest or an uncaring attitude. Apathy is very difficult to treat and requires a structured approach targeted at lifestyle, scheduling, and priority setting.

Traditional Therapies

Medications are rarely helpful in treating isolated apathy. Antidepressants, especially those that are more activating and non-sedating, can help when depression coexists with apathy. Similarly, acetylcholinesterase inhibitors used for dementia can help when cognitive problems coexist (see the next section on "cognitive decline"). Occupational therapy can help by reviewing goals, priorities, schedules, and strategies to help you deal with the effects of apathy. Other support individuals such as counselors, personal trainers, life coaches, and family members can help you stay on track with important tasks and goals.

Integrative Therapies

LIFESTYLE	SUPPLEMENTS	BODY	MIND-BODY	ENERGY	OTHER
Exercise*		Yoga	Meditation		Support Group
		Tai Chi			Pet Therapy
		Dance and Music			Nature Therapy
					Volunteerism

*Exercise can help through social engagement in treating depression and enhancing energy and confidence.

COGNITIVE DECLINE

Overview

Cognitive difficulties range from mild difficulty in finding words and trouble with multitasking to dementia, a condition in which thinking problems significantly impact daily function and independence. Cognitive problems can be caused by the disease, worsened by medications, and influenced by other problems such as depression and/or lack of cognitive and social engagement. Cognitive problems in PD are described as problems with executive function. Memory problems are not usually noted until cognitive changes are severe. Examples of executive dysfunction include difficulty with:

- Word finding
- Naming
- Multitasking

- Prioritizing and set-shifting (moving smoothly from one task to the next)
- Perceiving spatial relationships among objects (poor visuospatial skills)

Daytime sedation, apathy, depression, impulsive behaviors, and medicine-induced psychosis can also appear with cognitive changes. Psychosis is usually present in the form of visual hallucinations, but delusional thinking not based in rational thought can also occur.

Traditional Therapies

Treatment includes a multipronged approach that could include the following recommendations:

- Reduce medicines that can cause confusion if possible. These could include narcotic pain medicines, muscle relaxants, sedatives, and bladder antispasmodics.
- Change movement medicines. Focus on using dopaminergic medicines with a lower risk of cognitive problems and hallucinations such as rasagiline (Azilect®) and carbidopa/levodopa (Sinemet®) over those with a higher risk such as dopaminergic agonists, amantadine, and anticholinergics.
- Treat depression, anxiety, and sleep problems.
- Treat other medical problems including vitamin B12, vitamin D or thyroid deficiency, sleep apnea, infection, heart disease, diabetes, and dehydration.
- Add cognitive-enhancing medicines. Acetylcholinesterase inhibitors are medications that block the breakdown of acetylcholine in the brain, essentially increasing the levels of this neurotransmitter. Acetylcholine is an important neurotransmitter for cognitive and memory processes and levels are reduced in PD dementia.
- Treat hallucinations if necessary. Acetylcholinesterase inhibitors can improve mild hallucinations. Otherwise antipsychotic medicines may be needed. Most antipsychotic medicines can worsen PD movement symptoms so should not be used. Two agents are recommended to treat hallucinations: quetiapine (Seroquel®) and clozapine (Clozaril®).
- Refer to rehabilitation specialists, especially occupational therapy.
- Support the caregiver.

Integrative Therapies

LIFESTYLE	SUPPLEMENTS	BODY	MIND-BODY	ENERGY	OTHER
Foods	Coconut Oil	Yoga	Breath-work	Reiki	Support Group
Exercise*	Phosphati-dylserine	Tai Chi	Meditation	Acupuncture	Pet Therapy

(continued)

Integrative Therapies (*continued*)

LIFESTYLE	SUPPLEMENTS	BODY	MIND-BODY	ENERGY	OTHER
	Vitamin B12	Dance and Music	Guided Imagery	Bright Light	Music and Art Therapy
	Vitamin D	Massage	Biofeed-back	Aromatherapy	Volunteerism

*Exercise can help in many ways. High-intensity exercise is especially helpful for depression and cognition. Tai chi, dance, and yoga are exercises that place particular emphasis on the relaxation response.

CONSTIPATION

Overview

Neurologic problems with gastrointestinal control are noted early in the disease. This can include delayed gastric emptying with bloating or reflux, and reduced peristalsis and slowed movement of digested food through the small and large colon. Some medicines, especially anticholinergic medicines used to treat tremor or overactive bladder, and lifestyle changes can also cause constipation. Constipation can impede absorption of medicine and nutrients. Severity can range from mild discomfort to severe colon dilatation, leading to pseudo-obstruction. Pseudo-obstruction is caused not by a physical intestinal blockage but by a lack of normal peristalsis or intestinal movement. If untreated, this condition can lead to perforation, which is a medical and surgical emergency.

Traditional Therapies

Therapy includes a combination of diet, behavioral modification, and medication. These treatments are as follows:

- Medication review. Talk to your health care provider about certain medicines that can worsen constipation. They include amantadine and anticholinergic medicines used to treat PD motor symptoms and certain bladder medicines used to treat urinary urgency.
- Bowel training program. Occupational and physical therapists can help establish a bowel health program that includes scheduling time to use the bathroom each morning.
- Increase fluids and fiber in the diet.
- Use laxatives and stool softeners such as magnesium-based products, soluble fiber like Metamucil®, polyethylene glycol (Miralax®), and bisacodyl (Dulcolax®).

Integrative Therapies

LIFESTYLE	SUPPLEMENTS	BODY	MIND-BODY	ENERGY	OTHER
Water	Magnesium	Yoga	Biofeedback****		Walking/ Nature
Foods*	Probiotics	Tai Chi			
Exercise**	Ginger	Massage***			

*High-fiber foods include dried fruit (prunes and apricots), oats, whole grains, and fibrous fruits and vegetables such as leafy greens. Probiotic foods include yogurt, kefir, kombucha, pickled and fermented vegetables, sauerkraut, and senna tea. The recipe for fruit paste (following) is not only helpful for relieving constipation, but is also high in antioxidants.

**Walking is one of the best exercises.

***Abdominal massage can be performed on yourself using a gentle downward stroke or circular motion with the fingertips. Avoid abdominal massage if it is associated with pain.

****Physical and occupational therapists specializing in bowel and bladder control often have training in biofeedback.

Anti-Constipation Fruit Paste

1 pound pitted prunes

1 pound raisins

1 pound figs

1 cup brown sugar

1 cup lemon juice

1 tablespoon senna leaf tea (steeped in 2.5 cups water for five minutes and strained)

Add fruit to tea and boil for five minutes. Remove from heat. Add sugar and lemon juice. Blend to paste and store in freezer. Try freezing daily serving in ice cube tray. Use one to three teaspoons daily or as needed.

Easy Paste

Mix 1 cup bran, 1 cup apple sauce, and ¾ cup prune juice. Refrigerate. Use one to two tablespoons daily.

DEPRESSION

Overview

Depression can occur as a symptom of the disease, reaction to loss of abilities, or fear of change. It is also associated with other medical conditions common with aging or influenced by lifestyle changes such as lack of exercise or social engagement Depression could be generalized or experienced as a non-motor fluctuation (often experienced at end of dose). Anxiety often occurs with depression.

Depression can cause many symptoms beyond mood changes, including altered sleep patterns, appetite changes, apathy, fatigue, cognitive difficulties, and pain. Depression can significantly impact and limit participation in positive lifestyle changes and activities for health.

Traditional Therapies

These therapies usually include a combination of counseling (talk therapy) and medication. Cognitive behavioral therapy is a form of counseling. Cognitive behavioral therapy is a particularly helpful technique that helps identify negative thought patterns and habits that affect feelings and the decisions made each day. Awareness of these patterns of thoughts and actions is the first step in making change. Antidepressants are sometimes needed and often chosen based on the type of depression or other problems that may coexist with depression. SSRIs (e.g., sertraline, citalopram, escitalopram, fluoxetine, paroxetine) help mood, impulsivity, and anxiety. Others such as bupropion (Wellbutrin®) and venlafaxine (Effexor®) are more energizing and may be chosen when fatigue, energy, or apathy prevail. Still others are used to treat coexisting sleep problems or pain, such as mirtazapine (Remeron®) or duloxetine (Cymbalta®), respectively.

A medical examination can also identify other medical conditions that can worsen depression such as hypothyroidism, electrolyte abnormalities, anemia, heart disease, sleep apnea, and vitamin B12 and D deficiency.

Integrative Therapies

LIFESTYLE	SUPPLEMENTS	BODY	MIND-BODY	ENERGY	OTHER
Foods*	Tryptophan	Yoga***	Breath-work	Reiki	Support Group
Exercise**	Lavender, Lemon Balm, and Valerian Root	Tai Chi	Meditation	Acupuncture	Animal Therapy
	St. John's Wort (should not be used with Azilect)	Dance and Music	Guided Imagery	Healing Touch	Community Socialization
	Fish Oil	Massage	Biofeedback	Bright Light	Journaling
	Vitamin B12, Folate, B6, D	Feldenkrais Method® and Alexander Technique®	Hypnosis	Transcranial Magnetic Stimulation	Music and Art Therapy

(continued)

Integrative Therapies (*continued*)

LIFESTYLE	SUPPLEMENTS	BODY	MIND-BODY	ENERGY	OTHER
				Aroma-therapy	Prayer
					Nature Therapy

*Foods high in folate, B6, and B12 can reduce risk of depression.

**Exercise can help in many ways. High-intensity exercise is especially helpful when depression is also present. Tai chi, dance, and yoga are exercises that place particular emphasis on the relaxation response.

***A form of yoga called laughter yoga uses the power of laughter, group involvement, and body movement to enhance mood and well-being.

FATIGUE AND SEDATION

Overview

There are many potential causes of fatigue and daytime sleepiness. Daytime fatigue and sedation can result from a poor night's sleep or may be independent of sleep problems. Fatigue is a very common symptom of PD. Excessive movement (tremor or dyskinesia), reduced stamina or endurance, and the increased physical work of movement with PD can contribute to fatigue. Dopamine medicines, especially dopamine agonists. can cause excessive sedation and even sleep attacks. Other medicines such as antidepressants, anti-anxiety medications, pain medicines, and muscle relaxants can cause sleepiness (see the subsequent section on "sleep problems").

Traditional Therapies

It is important to reduce medicines that cause daytime fatigue when possible, including use of nighttime sleep medicines that cause daytime somnolence. Dopaminergic agonists may need to be reduced if they are associated with sedation, or sometimes increased if fatigue is noted as an end-of-dose problem. A search for other medical problems such as hypothyroidism, vitamin deficiency, poor diabetic control, dehydration, low blood pressure, sleep apnea, depression, and anemia should be completed and treated if present. Amphetamine-like stimulants are sometimes used, although their use is limited by side effects including hallucinations. A class of medicines that promote wakefulness are sometimes helpful. These include modafinil (Provigil®) and armodafinil (Nuvigil®). Finally exercise, physical therapy, and occupational therapy can help to increase stamina and strength, improve movement, and determine energy conservation strategies.

Integrative Therapies

LIFESTYLE	SUPPLEMENTS	BODY	MIND-BODY	ENERGY	OTHER
Foods*	Caffeine	Yoga	Breathwork	Reiki	Music and Art Therapy
Exercise**	Iron***	Tai Chi	Meditation	Acupuncture	
	Creatine	Massage	Guided Imagery	Bright Light	Aromatherapy****
			Biofeedback		Pet Therapy

*Foods low in glycemic load limit the rapid drops in blood glucose levels measured after ingestion and offer more sustained energy than simple sugars, processed carbohydrates, and high glycemic load foods. Avoid large heavy meals and eat smaller, more frequent meals instead.

**Aerobic exercise and resistance training can help reduce daytime fatigue.

***Iron supplements are only recommended when deficient.

****Peppermint and eucalyptus are examples of energizing essential oils.

NAUSEA

Overview

Nausea is a common side effect of all dopaminergic medicines. Some medicines such as dopamine agonists more commonly cause this problem. Gastric bloating, acid reflux, or delayed gastric emptying can contribute to nausea.

Traditional Therapies

Nausea can be minimized or avoided by starting medication at a low dose with a gradual increase in dosage as appropriate. Taking medications with food can also be helpful. Protein does interfere with the absorption of levodopa, so this medicine is usually prescribed with instructions to take without food. However, food (and water) can help buffer nausea when first beginning this medicine. Unlike many medicine-induced side effects, nausea often decreases over time.

Carbidopa can reduce the nausea associated with levodopa and, for this reason, is combined with levodopa (carbidopa/levodopa). Carbidopa blocks the metabolism or breakdown of levodopa prior to entry into the brain, minimizing nausea caused by these breakdown products. Extra carbidopa (25 mg) can be prescribed to be taken with standard carbidopa/levodopa dosing to further reduce nausea caused by levodopa.

Caution should be used when taking anti-nausea medicines since some work by blocking dopamine and therefore worsen PD motor symptoms. Examples of anti-nausea medicines to avoid include prochlorperazine (Compazine®), promethazine (Phenergan®), and metoclopramide (Reglan®). It is helpful to keep a list of your daily medicines with you at all times. Consider adding these medicines to the list under a separate category labeled "medicines to avoid."

Integrative Therapies

LIFESTYLE	SUPPLEMENTS	BODY THERAPY	MIND BODY	ENERGY	OTHER
Foods*	Ginger		Breathwork	Reiki	
	Licorice		Meditation	Acupuncture	
	Peppermint		Guided Imagery		
	Probiotics		Biofeedback		
	Chamomile, Lemon Balm				

*Small, more frequent meals can reduce gastric bloating and symptoms of reflux that can worsen nausea. Ginger-based foods, especially whole ginger and candied ginger, can help relieve nausea.

ORTHOSTATIC HYPOTENSION (DIZZINESS)
Overview
Orthostatic hypotension is described as light-headedness or dizziness when moving from a lying position to sitting or from sitting to standing. This problem is caused when normal neurologic reflexes do not respond to change in movement against gravity, causing a drop in blood pressure. Symptoms of dizziness can lead to problems with light-headedness, fatigue, imbalance, falls, neck pain, labored breathing, cognitive "dulling," and loss of consciousness when extreme.

Orthostatic hypotension is a symptom that can accompany PD and can be caused by medicines. PD medicines, especially dopamine agonists, amantadine, and anticholinergic agents used for tremor and bladder control, are common medicines used by people with PD that can lower blood pressure and worsen this problem. Orthostatic hypotension is worse with low blood pressure, dehydration, and anemia.

Traditional Therapies
A cardiology consultation may be needed to be sure heart or circulation is not causing low blood pressure. Blood work can detect contributing problems such as anemia. Nonmedical treatment includes compression stockings, elevating the head of the bed by 30 degrees, elevating legs when sitting, drinking extra fluids, and adding salt to food. PD medicines and other medicines are often changed to minimize this problem. Physical therapists and occupational therapists can provide exercises and safety precautions to reduce symptoms and increase safety. Medications to boost blood pressure include fludrocortisone (Florinef®), midodrine (Proamatine®), and droxidopa (Northera®).

Integrative Therapies

LIFESTYLE	SUPPLEMENTS	BODY	MIND-BODY	ENERGY	OTHER
Foods*	Caffeine	Yoga	Breathwork		Animal Therapy++
Exercise**	Licorice***	Tai Chi	Meditation		
Water	Tyrosine	Massage	Guided Imagery		
			Biofeedback		

*Drinking plenty of fluids and eating foods high in salt can help increase volume in blood vessels and increase blood pressure.

**Exercising calf and leg muscles is important. Isometric exercise (muscle contraction without movement) such as squeezing a ball in your hands and tightening feet, calf, and thigh muscles before standing can help. Avoid increased abdominal pressure while exercising, which can worsen orthostatic hypotension. Drink plenty of water when exercising.

***Licorice supplement can be used to increase blood pressure, but only under the supervision of your health care provider, as life-threatening electrolyte abnormality (low potassium) can occur.

++Animals can be trained to recognize dizziness and help buffer your fall.

PAIN

Overview

Pain has many causes and treatment will change with the type and cause of pain. Pain can be related to PD, other conditions aggravated by PD, and specific syndromes that occur more frequently with PD. Pain is worse in the setting of depression and can influence other symptoms such as sleep, anxiety, and exercise tolerance. Some of the more common causes of pain:

- Parkinson's pain, which is as an "off" related problem (usually noted at end of dose), dystonia, and rigidity
- Musculoskeletal pain, which is associated with arthritis and perhaps worsened by postural changes, rigidity, and dyskinesia that puts more stress on joints
- Pain from other conditions more common with PD, including depression, restless legs syndrome, leg swelling, and blood clots
- Nerve pain, which includes peripheral neuropathy and radiculopathy (pinched nerve).

Traditional Therapies

Treatment includes a combination of medication, exercise, and behavioral management. Over-the-counter pain medicines such as acetaminophen (Tylenol®), ibuprofen (Motrin®), and naproxen (Naprosyn®) are most commonly used. "Off" related pain usually fluctuates with PD medicine in that pain is worse at end of dose or in the morning when medicine effect is worn off. Treatment usually focuses on "smoothing out" the effect of dopaminergic medicines, much in the same way motor fluctuations are treated. Pain related to dystonia, rigidity, or muscle spasm can sometimes respond to muscle relaxants such as baclofen or tizanidine or botulinum toxin injections. Neuropathic pain caused by nerve injury can respond to some tricyclic antidepressants such as amitriptyline or nortriptyline or duloxetine (Cymbalta®) and seizure medicines such as gabapentin (Neurontin®).

Physical therapy is an important part of pain control focusing on joint range of motion, posture, improved body mechanics, and strengthening weakened muscles. Occupational therapy performs similar therapy with a focus on shoulder or arm pain and improved work ergonomics.

Integrative Therapies

LIFESTYLE	SUPPLEMENTS	BODY	MIND-BODY	ENERGY+++	OTHER
Foods*	Fish Oil	Yoga	Breathwork	Reiki	Music and Art Therapy
Exercise**	SAMe	Tai Chi	Meditation++	Acupuncture	
	Chondroitin and Glucosamine	Massage***	Guided Imagery	Vibration Therapy, TENS++++	
	Magnesium	Chiropractic+	Biofeedback	Magnetic Stimulation	
	GABA		Hypnosis		

*Pain is often associated with inflammation. An anti-inflammatory diet high in unprocessed fruits and vegetables and healthy omega-3 fatty acids and low in processed foods, simple sugars, saturated fats and meat can help.

**All forms of exercise can help pain, but only when tailored to the person and performed correctly. Exercise programs should be guided by physical and occupational therapy to avoid worsening of pain and injury.

***Aggressive massage will worsen pain caused by dystonia. Also remember to instruct your massage therapist to avoid shoulders, head, and neck if you have a DBS implant.

+Acupuncture, massage, and chiropractic therapy should avoid the upper body to avoid damage to DBS hardware.

++Mindfulness-Based Stress Reduction (MBSR®) is a specific program that originated to help people with pain. MBSR classes are often available through large medical centers or hospitals.

+++Energy therapies that use magnetic fields or electricity can interfere with deep brain stimulation (DBS) therapy.

++++A transcutaneous electrical nerve stimulation (TENS) unit is a small portable device that applies low level electrical stimulation to the skin over areas of the body that are painful. Stimulation blocks painful nerve messages to the brain reducing pain.

RESTLESS LEGS SYNDROME
Overview

Restless legs syndrome (RLS) is restlessness in legs or body especially at the end of the day or at times of inactivity, usually evenings, greatly affecting one's ability to sleep. Distressful symptoms are relieved by movement. RLS can be primary (not caused by other conditions) and sometimes hereditary or secondary and associated with problems such as PD, peripheral neuropathy, and iron deficiency. The connection between PD and RLS is further strengthened in that both conditions are associated with changes in dopaminergic regulations and improve with dopaminergic treatment.

Traditional Therapies

Medical therapies include dopaminergic medicines (similar to those used for PD motor symptoms), opioid narcotic agents, and other medicines used for nerve pain such as gabapentin (Neurontin®) and pregabalin (Lyrica®). Iron supplements can help in the setting of deficiency. A few words of caution:

- Be careful not to take certain sleep aids that can worsen RLS, such as diphenhydramine (Benadryl®) often found in over-the-counter sleep aids such as Tylenol PM® and Advil PM®.

- Avoid most antidepressants, some of which are used to help sleep. Bupropion (Wellbutrin®) is an antidepressant that does not worsen RLS.

- Avoid alcohol, caffeine, and stimulants at night.

Integrative Therapies

LIFESTYLE	SUPPLEMENTS	BODY	MIND-BODY	ENERGY	OTHER
Foods*	Iron and Vitamin C	Yoga	Breathwork	Acupuncture	Vibration Therapy+
Exercise**	Chamomile, Lavender, Lemon Balm, and Valerian Root	Tai Chi	Meditation	Reiki	Aromatherapy
	Tyrosine	Massage***	Guided Imagery	Vibration	
	Mucuna Pruriens		Biofeedback		

*Foods high in iron (meat, seafood, beans, molasses, dried apricots, and raisins) can help treat iron deficiency. Foods rich in magnesium and calcium can help muscle spasm and relieve the symptoms of RLS. Vitamin C (citrus, spinach) improves iron absorption.

**Gentle exercise such as stretching, yoga, and massage can help relieve discomfort. Aerobic exercise and resistance training can help nighttime sleep and decrease associated daytime fatigue.

***Massaging the legs at night can help reduce leg discomfort.

+Relaxis® is a medical device recently cleared by the Food and Drug Administration (FDA) and requires a prescription. A pad placed under the legs delivers 35 minutes of gentle vibration therapy to help RLS symptoms and aid sleep.

SLEEP PROBLEMS
Overview
Sleep problems range from trouble getting to sleep, trouble staying asleep, and early-morning awakening. Problems that can impact sleep include symptoms of pain, muscle spasm, dystonia, and tremor. Anxiety, depression, impulse control problems, nighttime hallucinations, confusion, and urinary frequency will also influence sleep. Unique sleep-related changes that can be associated with PD include restless legs syndrome, REM sleep disorder, sleep apnea, and fragmented sleep. Sedatives used to help sleep, although sometimes necessary, do bring side effects of confusion, daytime sedation, tolerance, and addiction.

Traditional Therapies
Therapies can be divided into behavioral changes (otherwise referred to as sleep hygiene), PD-specific treatments, and sleep medications. The following recommendations can help you get a good night's sleep:

Sleep Hygiene

- Go to bed and awaken at the same time each day to set up a habit.
- Keep your bedroom dark. Use nightlights if needed to illuminate steps to the bathroom.
- Limit computer use in the evening. Computers (and TVs) can affect sleep by keeping you up too late and engaging your mind in a way that you cannot "turn it off." In addition, lights emitted from monitors alter neuro-hormonal systems and circadian rhythms, tricking your brain into thinking that sleep should be delayed.
- Remove the TV from the bedroom.
- Avoid stressful situations before bed, such as watching the news or doing financial chores.
- Increase relaxing activities such as gentle stretching, yoga, and taking a hot bath.
- Drink the majority of your fluids before 5 p.m. if you awaken frequently to urinate ("urinary problems" are discussed in the next section).

Treat other sleep-related problems as well, including:

- Anxiety
- Depression
- Restless legs syndrome
- Confusion
- Vivid dreaming or hallucinations
- Sleep apnea
- Bladder control

Treatments for Muscle and Movement Control

- Reduce medicine off time and troublesome nighttime motor symptoms such as rigidity, tremor, and dystonia. Medicine wearing off can be worse at night and early morning especially if you do not take medicine between bedtime and the morning. Talk to your health care provider about medicine strategies that can increase medicine effectiveness throughout the night, such as the use of controlled-release preparations, agonists, and monamine oxidase (MAO) and catechol-o-methyl transferase (COMT) inhibitors.

- Reduce muscle spasms and dystonia through the following methods:
  - Use electric blankets for warmth.
  - Take magnesium and calcium supplements, which can help spasm.
  - Avoid dehydration and drink plenty of water during the day.
  - Ask your health care provider about botulinum toxin (Botox®, Myobloc®, Dysport®, and Xeomin®), which can reduce painful dystonia. An example is early-morning foot dystonia usually described as painful cramping of feet, toes, and calf in the middle of the night or morning.

Bed Comfort and Environment

- Try silk sheets and bedclothes that reduce friction, making turning in bed easier.

- Experiment with mattress types. Memory foam, waterbeds, or a soft mattress will make moving in bed more difficult. Extra firm mattresses can cause too much pressure on hips, shoulders, and elbows, causing numbness.

- Create a restful bedroom by using soothing colors, avoiding visual clutter, and playing soft music and nature sounds.

- Ask your doctor for a referral to an occupational therapist for other recommendations to help you more comfortably move and get in and out of bed.

Medications and Sleep Aids

Medications for sleep include:

- Benzodiazepines such as diazepam (Valium®), clonazepam, or lorazepam
- Sedatives such as zolpidem (Ambien®), eszopiclone (Lunesta®), zaleplon (Sonata®)
- Muscle relaxants, antipsychotics, antiseizure medications, and antidepressants such as baclofen, tizanidine, quetiapine, nortriptyline, amitriptyline, gabapentin, and trazodone are used for their sedating side effects when these other problems are also noted.
- Over the counter medicines often contain alcohol and antihistamines such as diphenhydramine (Benedryl®).

These medications can help sleep, but they do have additional risks or concerns. Many medications work better at improving sleep onset than preventing early-morning awakening, which is a bigger concern for most individuals. Additional concerns are:

- Excessive early-morning sedation
- Increased risk of falling
- Confusion, hallucinations, and vivid dreaming
- Tolerance
- Addiction
- Worsening of restless legs syndrome (especially if using certain sleep aids such as diphenhydramine or Benadryl® and certain antidepressants used for sleep)

Integrative Therapies

LIFESTYLE	SUPPLEMENTS	BODY	MIND-BODY	ENERGY	OTHER
Foods*	Tryptophan	Yoga	Breathwork	Reiki	Aroma-therapy
Exercise**	Chamomile, Lavender, Lemon Balm and Valerian Root	Tai Chi	Meditation	Acupuncture	Journaling
	Melatonin	Massage	Guided Imagery	Bright Light	
	Medical Marijuana		Biofeedback		
	GABA				

*Foods high in tryptophan along with carbohydrates are used for sleep promotion.

**Gentle stretching, yoga, or tai chi before sleep can help, while nighttime high-intensity exercise can impair sleep. Tai chi, dance, and yoga are exercises that place particular emphasis on the relaxation response. High-intensity exercise may be helpful when depression is also present.

URINARY PROBLEMS

Overview

Bladder problems are common, occurring in 20% to 50% of people with PD, caused by changes in the neurologic control of bladder function. The most common bladder problems include frequency of urination, urgency of urination, and excessive nighttime urination called nocturia. Other problems such as retention (difficulty emptying) can occur especially in men with an enlarged prostate or with certain medicines, including anticholinergics used for tremor and amantadine. Stress incontinence, described as incontinence after increased abdominal and pelvic pressure (e.g., during sneezing laughing, or jumping), is more common in women after childbirth or after pelvic floor surgeries. Urinary incontinence could also be a sign of a bladder infection.

Traditional Therapies

Since there are so many causes of incontinence, a urology evaluation that includes a urodynamic test (which measures bladder pressures before and after urination) can help determine the cause of bladder problems. Treatment sometimes includes medicines that relax the bladder wall to reduce excessive spasm and urgency. Most medicines are anticholinergics and can cause other problematic side effects such as memory problems, confusion, light-headedness, blurry vision, and constipation. A newer medicine with a different mechanism of action, mirabegron (Myrbetriq®), does not have this constellation of side effects and may be safer to use in the setting of low blood pressure or cognitive problems. Other medicines are designed to help prostate-related problems, retention, and bladder sphincter problems.

Physical and occupational therapists can help with bladder control and safety, especially given the risk of falls when rushing to the bathroom or when urinating at night.

Integrative Therapies

LIFESTYLE	SUPPLEMENTS***	BODY THERAPY	MIND-BODY	ENERGY	OTHER
Foods*	Cranberry		Breathwork	Acupuncture	
Exercise**	Saw Palmetto		Meditation		
			Guided Imagery		
			Biofeedback+		

*Cranberry juice is thought to help, but most brands have a low concentration of cranberry juice or are very high in sugar. Increasing fluids not only prevents dehydration but also reduces the risk of infection from unvoided urine in the bladder. Drink most fluids before 5 p.m. to limit nighttime urination.

**Kegel and other exercises can strengthen the pelvic floor.

***Cranberry supplements can reduce the risk of bladder infection especially in women prone to recurrent infections. Saw palmetto may improve symptoms of mild benign prostate hypertrophy in men.

+Physical and occupational therapy programs to treat incontinence often use biofeedback.

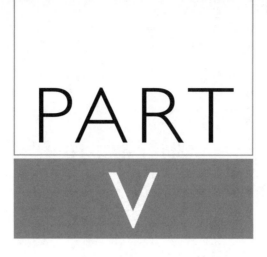

PART
V

Personalize Your Care

The following worksheets will help you develop an integrative health program that is right for you. Use them to guide your personal care plan. It may be helpful to bring them to your medical and therapy appointments for additional guidance and encouragement. All of the worksheets (except for the body mass index [BMI]) and the resources are available on my website, www.DrGiroux.com under the tab Brain Tools.

Organizing, Creating, and Sustaining Your Plan

Identifying what you need to do to improve your health and sense of well-being or to treat Parkinson's disease (PD) is just the first step. Understanding your degree of motivation, level of support to stay on track, and strategies to get you back on track when needed are the next steps. The following is designed to help you understand areas where you may need to focus or obtain more help.

How motivated am I to change? The following questions are designed to help you review whether your goal is backed by a true level of interest. Can your goal be modified to improve your motivation if interest is low?

- Is my interest in making healthy change strong, or am I following the desires of others?
- What would happen if I don't change?
- Do I believe these changes would make a difference?

What help do I have to change? These questions are designed to help you define your action plan. Are there steps that will work better for you?

- What are a few small steps I can take to move toward my goal?
- What obstacles or difficulties might stand in the way of my goal?
- What strengths can I capitalize on to begin change?

How will I stay on track? These questions are designed to help you stay on track or plan for how to get back on track.

- How will I keep up with my goal?
- Are there tools that can help me, such as websites, monitoring devices, or calendars?
- Can I partner with someone for support or guidance? For example, a life coach, counselor, friend, physical therapist, doctor, or trainer?

Personal Inventory

The best health care program is the one that is tailored to you. This survey will review your preferences, care philosophy, and current therapies to help you develop a balanced program and find the best programs and therapies based on your needs. Use this information to choose or change your treatment.

Balance

Using the following scale, answer each of the questions.

No	Disagree				Neutral			Absolutely Agree		
0	1	2	3	4	5	6	7	8	9	10

High Priority   Low Priority

Answer

Balanced Philosophy

I tend to focus on lifestyle over vitamins, supplements, and pills.   ____

I believe that holistic therapy is one that includes medicines when
needed.   ____

I believe that I can make a difference in how I feel or move.   ____

I believe natural therapies are not always better than traditional
medical therapies.   ____

Total   ____

These questions help you identify your thoughts about a holistic approach and its integration into traditional medicine. Your thoughts and ideas can stand in the way of an integrative approach. This is possible if you are resistant to traditional medicine, too skeptical of holistic medicine, or looking for a quick fix from natural therapies. With this in mind, reflect on how you answered the previous statements about a balanced philosophy. Add your answers together for your total score. If your score is 0 to 4, this is a high priority; if your score is greater than 7, this is a lower priority for personal reflection.

Balanced Lifestyle

I have taken steps to improve my diet.   ____

I have activities that help me manage stress.   ____

I have included exercise as part of my therapy at least three times week.   ____

My exercise program includes:

    Balance and posture exercise   ____

    Aerobic high-intensity exercise   ____

    Strength and flexibility exercise   ____

    Agility and motor learning (dance, tai chi)   ____

Total   ____

These questions help you identify lifestyle-related behaviors you are already doing or could benefit from adding to your routine. Add your answers together for your total score. If your score is 0 to 4, this is a high priority; if your score is greater than 7, this is a lower priority for personal reflection.

Analyze your answers to the preceding questions. The following questions will help you summarize your findings, what you have learned about yourself, and opportunities that exist for self-improvement.

Are your thoughts and current lifestyle balanced?

_____
_____
_____

What opportunities do you have to gain from this balance?

_____
_____
_____

Preference or Tendency
Circle the best answer(s)

I do better when I work . . .
Alone   In a group   Both

I prefer exercising . . .
At home   In a gym   Outdoors

I am . . .
Self-motivated
Need the help of a coach or buddy to stay motivated and keep going
Both

I tend to focus more . . .
On passive activities (e.g., massage)
On active activities (e.g., tai chi or meditation)
Both

I tend to do activities that . . .
Are in my comfort zone   Are new

Based on your answers, what activities would best fit these preferences or tendencies? Consider choosing a therapy or activity that is different from your usual tendency.

_____
_____
_____

Experience

Using the following scale, answer each of the questions that follow.

No	Disagree				Neutral			Absolutely Agree		
0	1	2	3	4	5	6	7	8	9	10
Low Priority								High Priority		

Answer

I have had little past experience with exercise, diet change or, stress management. ____

I rely on the stories of others to decide on a therapy rather than discussing them with my medical care team. ____

Total ____

These questions explore your experience with lifestyle change and how you make decisions about your care. Add your answers together for your total score. If your score is greater than 7, you may benefit from greater support and more guidance from trained professionals.

Based on your answers, do you think you would benefit from greater clinical guidance?

_____

_____

_____

Assembling Your Integrative Team

Physician Discussion Tool

Many doctors are skeptical about alternative and integrative therapies. You may find that doctors or health care providers are resistant to discussing these therapies with you, yet it is so very important to include them in your care decisions. This worksheet offers you tips or strategies that can help you talk with your doctor or health care provider about an integrative medicine therapy.

- **Begin by reinforcing your desire for a holistic approach.** State your desire to, ideally, include your doctor as a partner in this approach.

- **Describe the therapy.** Do not assume your doctor is aware or has knowledge about a particular therapy.

- **Define why a particular therapy is important to you.** For example, participation in a therapy can increase your sense of control or hope or create a feeling of holistic well-being and healing.

- **Identify your goal for therapy.** Examples of goals could be tremor control, stress management, pain relief, better sleep, or more energy.

- **Define how you will measure the success of a therapy.** Give thought to how long you will continue a therapy before deciding it is or is not effective.

- **Describe how this therapy will complement traditional medical therapy.** This is important as many doctors have had experience with patients avoiding effective therapies prescribed in clinic for less effective alternative therapies. Begin the discussion by exploring how these therapies can work together; this approach can help overcome resistance from your doctor.

- **Identify how you believe a therapy can help even when not proven.** For instance, relaxation and stress relief are a benefit of many therapies such as acupuncture, massage, and Reiki. Focus on these known benefits and not just the many claims that are often unsubstantiated.

Practitioner Checklist

These questions can help you decide if a therapist, trainer, or healing practitioner is right for you.

Experience

How many years of experience does the practitioner have?

How much experience does the practitioner have treating people with PD?

What training does the practitioner have?

Does training include formal education?

Are practitioners certified or licensed? (Your state medical board can help you identify if a license is needed.)

Are they working outside their scope of practice, such as recommending medicine changes in the absence of a medical degree?

Do they participate in ongoing continuing education?

Practice and Style

Are practitioners willing to schedule an educational meeting to discuss their treatment, philosophy, and style of care?

Is their treatment wrapped up in hype and marketing, or is there real science with outcomes to suggest benefit?

Do they listen to and include you in their treatment plan?

Will they send a treatment summary to your PD doctor?

General Health Tools

Antioxidant Food Shopping List

Antioxidants prevent or repair cell damage from oxidative stress, which is a biochemical by-product of cellular metabolism. Protect your body and your brain from oxidative stress by choosing foods rich in antioxidants.

- Try adding one new food item each week.
- Eat fruits and vegetables with different colors. You will benefit from a variety of stress-fighting antioxidants.

SUPER FOODS FOR NERVE CELL HEALTH

These foods are ranked highest in antioxidants in their categories:

Fruits: cranberries, blueberries, and blackberries

Vegetables: colorful beans (such as red), green leafy vegetables, and peppers

Nuts and seeds: pumpkin seeds, pecans, walnuts, flaxseeds, and hazelnuts

Protein: wild salmon and soy

Beverages: red wine and green tea

Make a list of four foods from the following list that you will add to your shopping cart this month. Try to choose foods you do not usually eat, as well as foods from different antioxidant groups.

1. _____
2. _____
3. _____
4. _____

Vitamin C (yellow, orange, red): green vegetables, tomatoes, strawberries, broccoli, citrus fruits and juices, apple juice, potatoes, kiwi, green-red-yellow peppers

Vitamin E: whole grains including brown rice, green vegetables, nuts, seeds, vegetable oils, wheat germ, papayas, avocados, sweet potatoes, peanut butter

Vitamin A (carotenoids, yellow and orange): sweet potatoes, carrots, tomatoes, kale, collard greens, apricots, cantaloupe, peaches, pumpkin, broccoli, pink grapefruit

Flavonoid (red, purple, blue): pomegranate, tea, soy, chocolate, black and kidney beans, grapes, wine berries

Selenium: eggs, garlic, chicken, fish, grains, wheat germ and bran, Brazil nuts, shellfish, beans

Lignans: flaxseed and oil (omega-3 fatty oils), rye, oatmeal, barley

(continued)

SUPER FOODS FOR NERVE CELL HEALTH
(continued)

Lycopene (red, pink): watermelon, grapefruit (pink), and tomatoes

Lutein (green): spinach, kale, broccoli, kiwi, Brussels sprouts, and other dark green vegetables

How can you estimate the antioxidant levels in your food?

The ORAC unit (Oxygen Radical Absorbance Capacity) is a measure of antioxidant activity in foods. This measurement system was developed by the National Institutes of Health (NIH). Learn more about superfoods and their ORAC units at www.oracvalues.com

Body Mass Index

Body mass index (BMI) is a measurement of weight, body fat, obesity, and health risk. The higher your BMI, the greater your risk of heart disease, stroke, dementia, diabetes, hypertension, and even cancer. BMI is calculated from height and weight according to the following formula:

$$BMI = Weight\ in\ pounds\ /\ (Height\ inches \times Height\ inches) \times 703$$

BMI <18.5	Underweight
BMI 18.5 to 24.9	Normal
BMI 25 to 29.9	Overweight
BMI >30	Obese

BMI is not perfect, because this index can overestimate body fat in athletes with high muscle mass and underestimate body fat in the elderly or people with low muscle mass.

Waist Circumference

Waist circumference, along with BMI, is used to screen for obesity-related disease risk. A waist circumference greater than 35 inches in women and 40 inches in men is associated with higher risk. Waist circumference is measured just above the hip bone at the level of the belly button after a normal expiration.

Other ways that obesity can affect PD include:

- Increasing fatigue and low energy
- Reducing stamina
- Producing shortness of breath
- Creating poor posture and balance, due to an altered center of gravity with increased abdominal fat
- Reducing PD-associated speech volume that can worsen because increased waist circumference increases upward pressure on the diaphragm, limiting volume of breath

Exercise Exertion and Maximum Heart Rate for Exercise

Investigating the effect of high-intensity exercise on PD, neuroprotection, and neuroplasticity is an important topic of research. There are many ways to quantify exertion. The following three strategies are practical ways to quantify exercise intensity. Discuss how to best rate your exercise intensity with your physical therapist or health care provider to avoid problems.

Talk Test

Mild Exertion: no change in speech

Moderate Exertion: can talk but not sing

Vigorous Exertion: can say a few words without pausing for breath

Pros: The talk test is very easy to use and understand. It is applicable to older people and individuals with PD since it does not rely on heart rate or age.

Cons: The test can be subjective.

Borg Perceived Exertion Scale[1]

This scale ranges from 6 to 20 and is based on a person's perception of exertion, or how the physical stress, effort, or fatigue of exercise feels. The higher the number the greater the exertion. When multiplied times 10, this number correlates with heart rate while exercising. For example a score of 9×10 = estimated exercise heart rate of 90.

Pros: The Borg rating is easy to use without the need for calculations.

Cons: It is not quantitative and is based on studies of males in their 20s, so may not apply to individuals with PD.

Percent Maximum Heart Rate

Moderate Exertion: 50% to 70% maximum heart rate

Vigorous Exertion: 70% to 85% maximum heart rate

Estimate of Maximum Heart Rate: 220 – Age = Maximum

Pros: Heart rate is not subjective and digital monitors such as wristbands can calculate this for you.

Cons: PD can be associated with a blunted heart rate to exercise. This means that heart rate does not increase appropriately with increased exercise intensity.

---

[1] Centers for Disease Control and Prevention, http://www.cdc.gov/physicalactivity/everyone/measuring/exertion.html

Lifestyle Tools

Exercise Inventory

Creating an exercise routine means planning your schedule, managing your time, and identifying strategies to keep you on track. Taking a few minutes to plan and commit to the challenge in writing is worthwhile since exercise is such an important part of your PD treatment. You can use this form to guide your discussions with your physical therapist, trainer, or health care provider.

Exercise Goal

CATEGORY	EXAMPLE	DAYS PER WEEK	MINUTES PER WEEK	SYMPTOMS
Aerobic, cardio, or high intensity (e.g., fast-paced walking, cycling, rowing)				
Balance/posture/motor control (e.g., yoga, tai chi, dance, non-contact boxing)				
Resistance and flexibility (e.g., yoga and weight lifting)				
Neuro-reeducation or sensorimotor integration (e.g., exercises that use all your senses: Feldenkrais Method®, dance, yoga, Big and Loud®)				
Personal meaning activities (e.g., that give enjoyment, inspire passion)				

Obstacles, Strengths, and Opportunities

Use the following tool to identify unique circumstances that influence your exercise routine and solutions to obstacles that stand in your way.

OBSTACLE	POSSIBLE SOLUTIONS
Apathy	__Exercise with a partner. __Use a health coach or physical therapist. __Post an exercise calendar on your fridge. __Give yourself a reward for exercise. __Join a group rather than exercising alone. __Other:
Pain	__See a physical therapist to guide your exercise program. __Select low-impact and mind-body exercises such as therapeutic yoga or aqua therapy. __Other:

(continued)

Obstacles, Strengths, and Opportunities (continued)

OBSTACLE	POSSIBLE SOLUTIONS
Balance Problem	__See a physical therapist to guide your program. __Try aqua therapy or chair exercises. __Other:
Stamina or Fatigue	__See a physical therapist to guide your program. __Start small, if even just a few minutes every day, and slowly build up exercise time and endurance. __Other:
Illness	__Change routine to simple exercises such as gentle stretching. __Other:
Too Busy	__Set a schedule each week. __Commit to even a few minutes each day rather than no exercise at all. __Park and walk; take the stairs. __Schedule small exercise breaks at your desk and in the office. __Other:
Weather	__Plan both indoor and outdoor routines. __Try exercises that take advantage of the changing seasons (walking in the park, swimming, snowshoeing). __Find CDs or online routines that can be done at home during bad weather. __Other:
Transportation	__Find CDs or online routines that can be done at home during bad weather. __Contact your community center to see if there are ride-share arrangements. __Work with your support group or community foundation to develop a ride-share program. __Other:

(continued)

Obstacles, Strengths, and Opportunities (continued)

OBSTACLE	POSSIBLE SOLUTIONS
Vacation/ Change Routine	__Find CDs or online routines that can be performed when away from home. __Call ahead to learn of exercise programs at hotel facilities or local gyms. __Other:
Don't Like Exercise	__Find fun and social activities such as boxing and dancing. __Walk in the park or outdoors rather than on a treadmill. __Other:
Other:	

Health, Diet, and Nutrition Survey

Do you have a personal habit or medical condition that could benefit from healthier eating? Are your eating habits optimized for brain health? Take this survey and learn where you can make a difference.

Medical Health

My weight is within a healthy range.

	Disagree									Agree
	0	1	2	3	4	5	6	7	8	9	10

I drink more than one glass of alcohol daily.

	Often									Never
	0	1	2	3	4	5	6	7	8	9	10

I smoke or chew tobacco.

	Often									Never
	0	1	2	3	4	5	6	7	8	9	10

I exercise four or more times weekly.

	Never									Often
	0	1	2	3	4	5	6	7	8	9	10

Medical conditions or symptoms I have that are also affected by diet. (Circle all that apply.)

Diabetes	High cholesterol	High blood pressure	Heart disease
Stroke	Ulcers	Intestinal problems	Constipation
Fatigue	Dizziness	Arthritis	Cancer
Depression	Anxiety	Dementia	
Parkinson's	Other brain disease	Acid reflux	

Priority for Change

Record your average scores for each category.

0 = Opportunity for Change

10 = Good Dietary Habits and Eating

Nutrition Knowledge _____

Eating Habits _____

Shopping and Cooking _____

Readiness for Change _____

Review your answers and you will learn where you must focus your efforts for better eating. Share this information with your health care provider to make it part of your treatment plan.

Do you have medical conditions that are affected by your diet? If so, how does this information affect your desire to change your diet and nutritional habits?

_____

_____

_____

Does this knowledge increase your desire to change your eating habits?

_____

_____

_____

Do you have the information or resources you need to eat better?

_____

_____

_____

Are there eating habits that you could change for better health?

_____

_____

_____

How could you change your shopping habits?

_____

_____

_____

How could you change meal planning and cooking?

_____

_____

_____

Are you ready for change?

_____

_____

_____

Nutrition Knowledge

I have a good understanding of healthy diet choices.

Disagree										Agree
0	1	2	3	4	5	6	7	8	9	10

I know the steps I need to take to eat better.

Disagree										Agree
0	1	2	3	4	5	6	7	8	9	10

I know how to read food labels.

	Disagree									Agree
	0	1	2	3	4	5	6	7	8	9	10

Average *Knowledge Score* (add scores and divide by 3) = _____

Eating Habits

I skip meals.

	Often									Never
	0	1	2	3	4	5	6	7	8	9	10

I read food labels.

	Never									Often
	0	1	2	3	4	5	6	7	8	9	10

I choose processed foods or fast food over fresh foods in their natural state.

	Often									Never
	0	1	2	3	4	5	6	7	8	9	10

I eat alone.

	Often									Never
	0	1	2	3	4	5	6	7	8	9	10

I take the time to enjoy my meals.

	Never									Often
	0	1	2	3	4	5	6	7	8	9	10

I eat while doing other chores or watching TV.

	Often									Never
	0	1	2	3	4	5	6	7	8	9	10

I eat when I'm stressed or bored.

	Often									Never
	0	1	2	3	4	5	6	7	8	9	10

I enjoy cooking or preparing food.

	Never									Often
	0	1	2	3	4	5	6	7	8	9	10

I stop eating when I'm full.

	Never									Often
	0	1	2	3	4	5	6	7	8	9	10

I binge eat.

	Often									Never	
0	1	2	3	4	5	6	7	8	9	10

I will usually try the latest new diet fad.

	Often									Never	
0	1	2	3	4	5	6	7	8	9	10

I drink sugary drinks or soda.

	Often									Never	
0	1	2	3	4	5	6	7	8	9	10

Average *Healthy Eating Score* (add scores and divide by 12) = _____

Shopping and Cooking

I choose organic foods when possible.

	Never									Often	
0	1	2	3	4	5	6	7	8	9	10

I use spices to flavor foods.

	Never									Often	
0	1	2	3	4	5	6	7	8	9	10

I read labels before purchasing food.

	Never									Often	
0	1	2	3	4	5	6	7	8	9	10

I tend to fry food and/or cook with fat.

	Often									Never	
0	1	2	3	4	5	6	7	8	9	10

I choose olive oil over dressings and spreads.

	Never									Often	
0	1	2	3	4	5	6	7	8	9	10

I buy/eat a variety of foods.

	Never									Often	
0	1	2	3	4	5	6	7	8	9	10

I plan my meals and shopping list in advance.

	Never									Often	
0	1	2	3	4	5	6	7	8	9	10

I buy locally from farmer's markets when possible.

        Never   Often

        0   1   2   3   4   5   6   7   8   9   10

I tend to buy convenience food, fast food, and prepared foods.

        Often   Never

        0   1   2   3   4   5   6   7   8   9   10

Average *Shopping and Cooking Score*
(add scores and divide by 9) = _____

Readiness for Change

I believe my food choices affect my health and well-being.

        Disagree   Agree

        0   1   2   3   4   5   6   7   8   9   10

I am ready to work on improving my food choices and habits.

        Disagree   Agree

        0   1   2   3   4   5   6   7   8   9   10

I am confident that I can make healthy eating changes or will seek help to do so.

        Disagree   Agree

        0   1   2   3   4   5   6   7   8   9   10

Average *Readiness for Change Score*
(add scores and divide by 3) = _____

Stress and Anxiety Inventory

Stress is a part of life. Stress can cause anxiety, which can become a chronic problem leading to excessive concern, preoccupation, and emotional distress. Physical problems worsened by chronic anxiety include problems with sleep, cognitive functions, mood, fatigue, digestion, appetite, headache, or pain, palpitations, and breathing problems. Use this worksheet to learn how stress affects your symptoms and take action. Be sure to talk with your health care provider about problems you are having with anxiety or stress and the potential treatment.

Stress Triggers. Keep a diary of when you feel the most stressed. Can you identify circumstances, activities, or times of the day that add to your stress or anxiety? List these triggers here.

1. _____
   _____
   _____
   _____

2. _____
   _____
   _____
   _____

3. _____
   _____
   _____
   _____

4. _____
   _____
   _____
   _____

Stress Symptoms. Think about how you feel when you are stressed or anxious. Does stress or anxiety affect any of the problems listed in the following? If so, describe the changes in your body or activity that occur.

Rate these changes on a scale from 0 to 10 (0 = no problem, 10 = most severe problem).

PROBLEM AREA	SEVERITY 0 TO 10	DESCRIBE PROBLEM, CHANGE IN ACTIVITY, OR BODY PART THAT IS AFFECTED. (USE SEPARATE SHEET IF NEEDED.)
Tremor		
Muscle tightness or spasm		
Speech or swallowing		
Stamina		
Sleep		
Trouble falling asleep		
Trouble staying asleep		
Fatigue		
Exercise or activity changes		

(*continued*)

Stress Symptoms (continued)

PROBLEM AREA	SEVERITY 0 TO 10	DESCRIBE PROBLEM, CHANGE IN ACTIVITY, OR BODY PART THAT IS AFFECTED. (USE SEPARATE SHEET IF NEEDED.)
Nausea, indigestion, change in appetite		
Dizziness, palpitations, or sweating		
Pain or headache		
Cognitive difficulties such as trouble concentrating, remembering, or focusing		
Emotional changes such as depression, negativity, hopeless-ness, or sense of doom		
Social activities such as withdrawal or decreased engagement in activities		

Calculate your stress impact scale by adding your answers above and dividing by 15: _____. (0 = no impact and 10 = significant impact.) Based on your answers, does stress play a role in your symptoms or overall well-being?

Stress Reduction. What changes are you already making to reduce stress? Think about what helps you deal with stress and write down what has worked for you.

_____

_____

_____

_____

_____

_____

Have you tried counseling, meditation, yoga, guided imagery, or deep breathing exercises?

Yes   No

How can you add these relaxation strategies to each day?

_____

_____

_____

_____

Exercise: Describe your exercise routine on an average week.

_____

_____

_____

_____

_____

What steps can you take to reduce your stress with exercise?

_____

_____

_____

_____

Resources

For the worksheets included in this book as well as more helpful tips to support better living with Parkinson's disease, visit www.DrGiroux.com. Worksheets are located under the Brain Tools tab.

NATIONAL PARKINSON'S FOUNDATIONS

American Parkinson Disease Association, www.apdaparkinson.org
Brain Stimulation Foundation, www.brainstimulationfoundation.org
Davis Phinney Foundation, www.davisphinneyfoundation.org
Michael J. Fox Foundation, www.michaeljfox.org
National Parkinson Foundation, www.parkinson.org
Parkinson's Action Network, www.parkinsonsaction.org
Parkinson's Disease Foundation, www.pdf.org

DEEP BRAIN STIMULATION

Deep Brain Stimulation Insights, www.dbsprogrammer.com

Acknowledgments

Many people have contributed to or made this book possible. First and foremost, I am thankful to the thousands of patients I have treated over the years. Their inspirational stories and courage in the face of challenge has taught me more about Parkinson's than all my formal training combined. I was fortunate to have had Jerrold Vitek, MD, PhD, Raymond Watts, MD, and Mahlon DeLong, MD, as mentors during my early years while a clinical fellow in movement disorders. I learned so much about the treatment of Parkinson's under their tutelage but it was their compassion for their patients that most shaped my own clinical approach and style of care. I also wish to acknowledge Gladys Gonzalez-Ramos, PhD. Although her life ended too early, her memory looms large as I remember the many conversations we shared in which she encouraged me to lead with the heart and explore a broader integrative approach to medicine. Ruth Hagestuen, RN, expanded my knowledge and appreciation of interdisciplinary care. Many foundations have given me the platform to share my clinical expertise in the field of integrative and wellness care, including the Davis Phinney Foundation, Michael J. Fox Foundation, National Parkinson Foundation, Northwest Parkinson's Foundation, and World Parkinson Congress.

I wish to thank the many experts that contributed to this book, including Theresa Ellis, PhD; David Leventhal; Maya McNeilly, PhD; Laurie Mischley, ND; Barbara Morgan, MD; Karl and Angela Robb; and Adam Simmons, MD. Each of these individuals has a unique perspective and I have benefited greatly from their collective knowledge, expertise, and wisdom. My sister, Michelle Zarrella, BS, RN, can be credited for helping me bridge the gap between science and application of these principles to everyday life and Renee Giroux reminds me of the possibilities that can grow when you pursue your passion. I wish to thank Demos Medical Publishing and editor Julia Pastore for believing in this project and the information it contains. Finally, I am especially grateful to the help and encouragement I have received from Sierra Farris, PA-C, MS. She contributed to this book in so many ways beyond sharing her expertise in DBS therapy and medical illustration. My work in the Parkinson's community would not be where it is today without her expertise, compassion, knowledge, and encouragement.

Index

About the Author

Monique L. Giroux, MD, is a practicing neurologist, author, and motivational speaker. She embraces a holistic approach to Parkinson's care including medical, surgical, rehabilitative, and integrative therapies, with a focus on treating the person not just the disease. Dr. Giroux's training is unique. She is fellowship-trained in both movement disorders and integrative medicine. Her informative blog, unique with its focus on self-care and holistic brain health, educates people internationally. She has experience and leadership in interdisciplinary care and extensive training in deep brain stimulation management, botox therapies, and mindfulness-based therapies.

Her practice, Movement & Neuroperformance Center of Colorado, is located in Englewood and Fort Collins.

www.drgiroux.com